Dear Cassidy

Thank you for just
being there ♡

Love,

Lisa Schofield
JMS
BC ...

Born Schizophrenic is a semi-sequel to *January First* by Michael Schofield. It continues their story up through early 2017, but it also covers the earlier years from Susan Schofield's perspective.

Born Schizophrenic: A Mother's Search for Her Family's Sanity

Susan Schofield

1. Non-fiction-Parenting & Relationships-Special Needs
2. Health, Fitness & Dieting-Mental Health-Schizophrenia

Paperback ISBN: 1544672314
Paperback ISBN-13: 978-1544672311

Printed in the United States of America

DEDICATION

For my babies, Jani and Bodhi Schofield. You brought me closer
to God than I could ever have imagined. ❤

TABLE OF CONTENTS

TABLE OF CONTENTS

FOREWORD

Like many mothers, I first met Susan Schofield in the pages of her then-husband Michael's 2013 book *January First: A Child's Descent into Madness and her Father's Struggle to Save Her*. I found Michael's book shortly after I shared my own family's struggles with parenting a son who had mental illness in a viral essay entitled "I Am Adam Lanza's Mother." That essay expressed my frustration and grief at a fragmented and broken mental healthcare system when my family's personal tragedy intersected with the very public tragedy of the Newtown school shootings

Unlike Susan and Michael, for many years I did not have the courage to put my name on our family's story. Instead, my family—and my sweet son—suffered, as so many other families suffer, in shame and silence. After Newtown, when my son's caseworker recommended that I charge him with a crime so that he could get access to much needed medical services for his biologically based brain difference, something in me broke. I put my name on my story.

Later, Eric ("Michael" in my essay and follow-up book *The Price of Silence: A Mom's Perspective on Mental Illness*) claimed his own story in a brave and beautiful TEDx Boise talk, where he explained what it was like to grow up in fear—of himself. Together, Eric and I now advocate to end our society's stigma and discrimination against people living with mental illness and their families.

Both my son Eric and the Schofield's children are testaments to the power of finding the right diagnosis and treatment. With the right treatment, there is hope. Recovery is possible. Every child—every family—deserves that chance.

I felt then and still feel now that the Schofields were very brave to share the details of their struggle to obtain a correct diagnosis and effective treatment for their daughter's child-onset schizophrenia. Like the Schofields, I faced the scorn of antipsychiatry adherents, the diffidence of overworked healthcare workers, the frustration of ignorant educators, and the painful avoidance of pretty much every other mom on the playground. When your child has a mental illness, it seems like everyone has the same unhelpful theory: blame the parents.

Born Schizophrenic picks up the story of Jani and her brother Bodhi, who also likely lives with schizophrenia, in their mother's words. The book is an unflinching and honest account from Susan's perspective of challenges that will feel familiar to far too many parents in America. As I read her words, I was struck by how many of the heartbreaking stories in Susan's life were similar to my own.

Both Michael and Susan have been criticized for living their family's life very much in the public eye. Is their story messy? Of course. Are they perfect parents? No parent is. But this story is important precisely because it's real. This raw glimpse into parenting special needs children will help others to better understand and empathize with us. Even the painful end of their marriage, which Susan repeatedly stresses was in no way Jani's or Bodhi's fault, highlights the extreme stresses that lack of access to affordable and effective healthcare can create in a family who just wants what any family wants: to be happy.

To say that "mental illness is not a casserole illness" is an understatement.

I am personally grateful to both Michael and Susan for allowing other parents to find a community by sharing their family's stories.

I am grateful for their courage in fighting to end the stigma of mental illness. And I am grateful to them both for their unfailing love for their very special children. I hope that Jani and Bodhi will add their voices to the story as they continue to work on their recovery.

And I hope that policy makers will read this book. A 1999 report from the National Alliance on Mental Illness entitled "Families on the Brink" outlined the critical shortages of care and compassion that families parenting a child with mental illness faced. Those challenges—both in care and compassion—still exist today. By sharing her family's story, Susan Schofield is helping all of us to understand that families don't need our judgment or our ignorance. All children deserve love.

Liza Long, Ed.D.
Author, "I Am Adam Lanza's Mother" and *The Price of Silence: A Mom's Perspective on Mental Illness* from Plume Press
www.lizalong.com

PREFACE

The World Health Organization (WHO) defines *Schizophrenia* as a severe mental disorder characterized by a profound disruption in thinking which affects language, perception, and the sense of self. Symptoms can include auditory and visual hallucinations as well as delusional thinking. *Autism* is a spectrum disorder centered around difficulties in communication and social interaction, and repetitive areas of interest and activities.

When our daughter January (Jani is her preferred name) was diagnosed with child-onset schizophrenia at six, the dreams my husband Michael and I had for our family's future became delusional, much like the illness itself. Our toddler son, Bodhi, was our shining hope at the time, a savior for his sister. He would be the one to look after Jani when we were no longer around.

This was not to be.

At two, Bodhi was diagnosed with autism and began to decompensate even with the best early intervention therapy, Applied Behavioral Analysis (ABA). Ironically, Jani started showing signs of improvement around the same time. Unlike her brother, she was finally on the right medications and therapies. This left us wondering if Bodhi had schizophrenia too.

Born Schizophrenic is a semi-sequel to my ex-husband Michael's book *January First*. It follows my journey as a special needs' mom trying to keep our family together as it's falling apart. *January First* was told through Michael's voice, but this is through mine. We are farther along Bodhi's journey now, shedding a new light and perspective on why it was so important that God gave us January first.

Susan Schofield
Valencia, California
May 1, 2017

ACKNOWLEDGMENTS

To my Mom and Dad (Lorraine & Ron), you've been my most vital support, both emotionally and financially as I've matured.

To Papa Abe and Grandma Rae, my Mom's parents who were there for me growing up. And most importantly, the side of my family no one really talked about. We saw them every so often but there was a hidden history with few pieces revealed. These were my Dad's parents, Grandma Freda, Papa Joe, and the uncle I never got to see, and neither did my father.

Maurice Mendlin died before his 4th birthday. He was a quiet, impulsive runner who was left alone in the kitchen one day as Grandma Freda and Great-Grandma Sophie were in the living room talking. The story passed down was that my Grandma Freda and her mother, Sophie, could not save him after he caught fire.

Later, Sophie encouraged my Grandma Freda to have another child. His name is Ron Mendlin and he is my father. Someday, I will tell his story as well. Grandma Freda was in and out of mental hospitals where she received electric shock treatments for depression. Her brother, Henry Kaufman, had schizophrenia and was institutionalized at the Napa State Hospital in California most of his life.

Genetics are truly amazing.

Cory Cabana, you are a Godsend! My dear friend from high school, Melinda Rockwell Burnside, sent you to me after guiding me through an unexpected divorce. Melinda, you gave me back my lost independence and Cory. I look forward to building a new foundation of love from which we'll grow. ♡

Uncle Harold, thanks for your visits and taking care of Friday's grooming needs. Dogs are expensive, especially the furry ones ☺ All the best to my niece, Jenne, who I'd like to think I talked into becoming a veterinarian at three, because she's a Sagittarius and that IS a likely career choice. She's in vet school as I write. Hope, your light is just beginning to shine!

Honey Doggie, my guiding light. You came as an angel in the night, teaching me never to give up on what seems impossible at the time. Friday, you're the best dog on Earth. We found you at the shelter at the right time. Honey would never have allowed caregivers and therapists in our home. We're lucky to have you. Ryder, you're our faithful bearded dragon, sitting on Jani's chest as we read the Bible at night.

Carl and Mary Goss, thank you for being "The Princess of Calalini's Benefactor." We appreciate all the help you've given us through the years. ♡ Dena Gittisarn, having been Bodhi's behaviorist since he was two and seeing everything I did, you validate me.

Ron, Grace, and Michi Rolek. I'm grateful for all your help and still use your book *Mental Fitness* to keep me "Calm in the Middle of the Storm." Jeanne, Lauren, and Joey Nicolosi, thanks for always being there. Angie Lussier, you and Hannah were a gift to Jani and me when no other friends were around. Pamela Malone Bernstein and your sons, Miles, Joel, and Shaun you have opened up your home to us since 2010 and I cannot thank you enough for all the help you gave. ♡ Lindsay Rickis, you have made every Christmas special for us, sending us boxes of better clothes than I could pick out for my kids. You are beautiful inside and out. Karlee Weston Corwell & Chelsee, your artwork is beautiful and decorating Jani's room. ☺

The Olive Garden, California Pizza Kitchen, and Red Lobster

make our kids feel comfortable during both good and especially "bad times." Plus, the play areas that welcome our kids: Sky High Sports, Scooters Jungle, MB2 Raceway, We Rock the Spectrum, Jump 5150, and the Fairfield Inn by Marriott Santa Clarita for our Jani Foundation "Halloween Rocks" events with magic by Rob Rasner at Rasner Magic Enterprises.

Sharone Rosen, I miss you being so close. I still need a good chiropractor. And, Dominic Garcia, you took the most beautiful picture of me EVER! I want to be "that girl" and for that moment in time, I was. I look forward to seeing you both at the wedding. ♡ You, too, Bonnie Keith of Video Magic Productions, along with David Jay of David Jay Entertainment for your Dee-Jaying 😊

Finally, a huge "Thank You" to all of you who donated to my Go-Fund-Me account when Michael left.

Special Recognition

Liza Long, thank you for writing an amazing Foreword to this book. I have an enormous amount of respect for your viral blog. "I am Adam Lanza's Mother." You were her voice and spirit.

Hadassah Foster, CEO/Founder of H&H Associates USA, speaks softly but carries a big stick. Christina Haselbusch (SKIP), you introduced me to The Real Life Church that accepts all our kids! Erin and Bruce Wilson, for your wonderful work with "If I Need Help," that provides wearable ID links to live profiles.

Valleri Crabtree, I support your political ambitions from the LGBT community to the Mental Health Community! Alex Blankenship, you give your mothers', Sherry Blankenship and Valleri, a right to be so proud. You will have a huge impact, whatever you do!

Stacey Cohen, you made the first call to Shari Roan at the LA Times back in 2009. This led to our meeting Gerri Shaftel, who has remained a "Constant" friend in the news department. Claire Weinraub and Elissa Stohler from 20/20 came out, then Dr. Phil and Discovery/TLC. Oprah, our Messenger, lead the pack with her producer, Erica Wohlreich, giving us a voice for those who could not speak to the current mental health care system in the United States, where those afflicted with schizophrenia are slipping on the yellow brick road, only to fall, waking up dead, or in prison.

Jennifer Hoff, you continue to fight for your son trapped inside psychosis and jailed with the word "Crazy" tattooed on his forward. Your funding behind the Jani Foundation is helping the parents of the new kids' coming, treating them to free fun-filled family events in safely enclosed environments. Laura Pogliano, you lost your son, Zac, to what mental illness can manifest into, suicide. This kind of grief will never go away, but you choose to fight for others with your own foundation, "Parents for Care." Angie Geyser & Morgan, you have been victims of what unrecognized mental illness can lead to and refuse to give up the fight for justice. There is hope with the new generation coming. Eli and Ruben, keep reaching for your goal to help kids who suffer from autism and mental illness.

Ron Thomas and Mary Sheldon, I am forever in Kelly's Army. Ron, your suffering was one of the worst in America's history, witnessing your son with schizophrenia, cry out for his Dad and God as he was being brutally murdered by Fullerton police officers in broad daylight. Then, to see those officers, acquitted. On July 5th, 2011, Kelly Thomas was viewed all over the world, being accused of a crime he didn't commit, then trying to understand the questions being fired at him by unruly police officers. Night-Sticks and Tasers brought him to an untimely, torturous death.

The Santa Clarita Police Department and the Department of Child & Family Services (CPS). I have been fortunate enough to meet you on so many occasions, good, and bad, but I'm grateful you know my kids... And they know you! Hopefully, this will make a difference as they grow up.

And lastly, to UCLA & Henry Mayo Hospital, as much as I am frustrated by "the system," AKA "The Game," I know you have to play it. Unfortunately, we ALL know that the insurance company lobbyists buy off our Representatives who allow insurance companies to make more money denying necessary treatment to mentally ill kids and adults; thus, creating collateral damage from Columbine to Sandy Hook. That said, while doctors fight insurance companies, social workers sink into a system set up to fail, leaving it up to us, the parents of mentally ill/autistic kids and adults to fight for them.

WORK ACKNOWLEDGMENTS

A huge thank you to my editor, Liz Long (POV Press). You helped me see what needed more explanation for an audience beyond myself.

Jacquelyn Mitchard, author of "Deep End of the Ocean," taught Michael and me writing techniques at the 2006 Maui's Writers' Conference, where we also met our friend, John Fetto. Thanks, Byrd Leavell (Waxman Leavell Agency) for your guidance through the first drafts of this book and your work selling *January First: A Child's Descent into Madness and Her Father's Struggle to Save Her*.

KFI, the best job EVER! I had so much fun working in talk radio during the 90s, so thank you David G. Hall, Mark Austin Thomas, Bill Handel, Marilyn Kagan, Dan Mandis, Gary Hoffman, Nick Federoff, John & Ken, Johan Beckles, Faith Beth Lamont, Joe Crummey, Scott Hasick, Casey Bartholomew, Rene Dominguez, Michael Crozier, Aida Murphy, and the Late Scott Greene. We had so much fun on "the night shift." A special thank you to Tony Dinkel and his son Anthony for being there during the hardest times with Jani and the early days when Bodhi was first diagnosed as autistic with intermittent explosive disorder.

KOST and KACE were in the same building as KFI. I found Karen Sharp (my first internship in radio, "Love Songs on the Kost"), Stella Prado Kuipers, Bryan Simmons, Ted Ziegenbusch,

Mark Wallengren, Kim Amidon, Fred Wallin, Dave Skyler, and Johnny Morris. Lisa Osborn, you helped me get my first on-air traffic job and Radene Marie Cook, you brought me to Metro Networks where I learned to report the news. There, I met Bill Thomas and trained with Colleen Spence who was in my Moms' Group as we were preggers at the same time. Twice! Here's a shout-out to Cole, Aubree, and Tom Spence of KVTA.

Judy Levitow, you advised us to have Honey smell Jani's clothing before meeting her. ♡ And of course, Jane Monreal, Gianna Suter, Geoff Peters, Eric Frost-Barnes, Mark Keene, Sandy Wells, Jack Savage, Phil Nash, Barry Turnbull, Lew Stowers, and Jennifer Marvin. I remember all the fun political conversations with Allen Lee. ☺ I vicariously went to Vegas, Friday night and came back Sunday morning, hitting the airwaves over the phone with Cory Baker and Tyrone Dubose on FM 98 & 99!

Metro did traffic and news through the IFB for KABC, KNX & KFWB. And, Denise Fondo, Tracie Savage, and Steve Kindred. Steve Truitt was at Metro too. He introduced me to Tracy Metro and "Born Schizophrenic." Tracy, Greg Spring, Ivy Brown, and Barry Gribbon all worked on it. Tracy introduced me to Elayne Howitt and the late Mike Simonoff, who took care of Jani and Bodhi.

Then there's Sharon Dale and Lucie Hill, who formed their own show on LATalkradio.com. We met up again when I hosted Bipolar Nation Radio there with my main co-hosts Vinny Wolf and Bert Hamaoui. Bert married Aylene Hamaoui and now they have three children!

Thank you, Sam Hasson, Dina Berkovich, and Ronin for giving me the opportunity to host Bipolar Nation. It was my therapy during the rockiest time in my life. Sheena Metal was there too. Psychic Linda Salvin came on as a guest and gave me a heads up on what was to come in my life. For more on my radio family, you can always seek out Don Barrett (@barrettLARadio). Also, watch for the cartoon about a special needs boy, "Little Billy," written and based on the life of the Simpsons' Lead Animator, Chance Raspberry.

FINAL ACKNOWLEDGMENTS

Western Bagel: Julie Sands and your daughter Amanda, at Tranquility, who did my hair for the wedding. Thank you. Also, the other Amanda who watched Bodhi grow as a baby and finally got a baby of her own, Brooke Mandy. You were always special to us. Doug, a regular, I always enjoy our conversations about the world. Plus,Zoe, Andrea, Sandra, Kyle Jennifer, Brayden and little Finnegan Schiner :) Of course, I can't leave out Francisco, always there to share your smile, as is Douglas, Nancy, McKenna, Johnny, Jeff, and Zoe. In the past, there was Gary, Stephanie and her daughter Joelle (she's going to be a psychologist... thank God she knows my kids)! And travelling further back into the past, I can never forget "Stan the Man" who passed away when Jani was 4. She still remembers how you played along with her and "90 the Firefly."

Also, the restaurants who've accepted our kids with open arms, The Olive Garden, California Pizza Kitchen, and Red Lobster.

Tim from AT&T and his wife, who support young adults let out of the system with nowhere to go after eighteen, mentally ill or not. Out of the goodness of their hearts, they give them food, shelter, and help finding a job. Tim, you are Golden.

My Moms' Group: Before all of this, we did everything together: Kim, Jessica, Kelly, Colleen, Lisa, Leah and of course, Bethanne. And then came, Jennifer Whitlock and Issac, who, although we lost touch did get at least some of Jani's "imagination."

Then came a new group, starting with Tracy Cooper & Matt. You gave me comfort on my very first run at this hospital game. Danae Eskildsen & Jason, Lisa Campos, Britt Kemp, Lisa Reinstein, Adrienne Carney & Lorna, Vanessa Rutherford, Alexa Norwood, Stephanie Garrison, Joyce Thomas, Kyle Marquez, and Amanda Herrington.

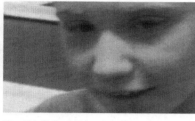

Bodhi Schofield. Abril 2017.

The doctors: Amelia, Ruth, Jessica, and his current outpatient psychiatrist who is still fighting for Bodhi to get an inpatient trial at UCLA, but still being denied by Dr. Hyde. Dr. Cam tried every-thing to convince Dr. Hyde and Danielle to treat him with Clozaril. Dr. Hyde waved him off leaving Dr. Cam to sigh, "There's nothing more I can do for him."

Melissa Spring Curras, Shelly Gummerus, Wendy Posey Songy & Ryan, Natalie Andrade Jonsson & Delicia, Jennah Tinajero & Jake, Lisa Gainer & Skylinn, Amanda Cooper Grimes & Justyce, Kelly Lyons Schaffer, Dawn Terry Stribling. And, a blue butterfly to Karen & the late Alysha Dunning.

My life support past and present: Carlos Rincoln, Parris, Ro-sario & Laura Martinez, Noah, Angie, Sara Estrada, Zachary Farmer, and many more behaviorists and caregivers who've come through our doors.

North of what was to become Silicon Valley, there was a suburb south of San Francisco named San Mateo County. We lived in Fiesta Gardens where I grew up with: the Hansons, Jon, Michele, and Laura Gault, Sandy Takayoshi-Berta, Joanna Malcom Cardinale, Bri-an Corcoran, Michelle Hamilton, Dena Derenale-Betti, Kathy Hall, Patricia Ellis Holt, Nader Nadershahi, Gale Ann Heiberger, Renee Walton, Cindy West, Debbie Bohan, Ryan and Zane Edwards, Cin-dy and Scott Dutra, Jack, Jeff and Jason Salvato, Lori, David, and Bette Levy, Carlos and Laura Ruiz-Early Gapinski, Mike Russell, and close neighbors Ernie & Mike Roeder. Amy Gonzales Bloom and Nancy Gonzales Beauchane were there, along with Stacey Thompson Alioto. Across the street, Norm, Betty, Brett, Sherry, and Kirk Henderson. (Your family holds an extra special place in my heart today.) Renee Rossi Hanke and the late Tony Rossi.

Just a few blocks from Fiesta Gardens, many of us went to Borel Middle School: Stefanie Aarons, Sity Schwartz, Noa Appleton, Sarah Hurd Montgomery, Paige Fallis, Paige McDonald, and Paige Morway Sullivan, Andrea Hornickle, Elena del Campo, Brad Wong, Andrea Marsala, and Lisa Cash.

Then we continued to Hillsdale High School: Lisa Breitenstein, Gracie Redmond, Kimmie Quan, Shelly Sibold Childers, Holst, Mark Friedman, Lissette Chacon-Villafan, April Smith, Tonya Fifield-Carter, Karen Campo Moore, Irene Harris, Laura Murray, Greg Baldwin, Vince Nubla, Andrew, Michelle, and Rebecca Gross. Robin Harris, Joyce, Erik & Stacey Martineau, Vince Aiello, Timothy Foley, Walter Chao, Rob Muchmore, Tom Minto, Andrea Hornickle, Carl Smith, Lennon Lansdown, Frank Wesley Rascue Quattlebottom, Monica Quintero-Devlaeminck, Mike Minnick, Sean McCarty, Bridget Baer Michelson, Diana Flores, Jane Lucas Tucker, Tracy da Silva Kirsten, Tracy Lerza Heiden, Sandra Tracy, Lori Dinatale, Spiro & Manuel-Manoli Tsingaris, Donna Van Aken Blevins, Michelle Atno-Hall, Lara Ervin, Cathy Van Noland, Cathy, Jason LaFlesch, Garth Bell, Kimberly Augustine, Kerri Brown, Shelly Armstrong, Shannon Soria, Marina Afanasieff, Tabetha A Stoner Revetta, David Draper, Roger Gauvreau, Barbara Bobbi Frew, Kelly Shannon, Colette Collum, Garth Bell, Jason Fritz, Doug Briggs, Jeff Kwan, Loretta Li, Ron Holst, Turner Morgan, Tom, Brandi, and Jen Mays, Gary & Anne Lundgren, Bridget Folan & The Bisconer Family, and the late Lori Pasqualino and Frank Datzman. Also, to Ara Bezjian and Egan Kingston for their work at The Stay Foundation.

My Facebook Family: Jessica Palumbo, Nicole Colbry, Josefine Miller, Zoey Roberts, Fred Stasek, Marie Bunn, John Lourenco, Vi-

FINAL ACKNOWLEDGMENTS

jay Pereiri, Taralynn Taylor, Melissa Wickstrom Sirek, Lea Stern Edgecomb Stetson, C. Christian Anderson, Lisa Perez Sullivan, Tremayne Kendrick Mosely, Melissa Seguin, David Todd, Matthew Robbins, Roko Karan, Joseph Eric Rajesh Janvier, David Reineke, Bill Grove II, Joe Miller, Roy Ferry, Caroline Lopez, Lorraine Waite, Cary Tobaben, Kathryne Sergent-Fisher, Sam Halabi, Biswajit Mukherjee, Nyoka Brooks, Sarasi Singh, Sondra Williams, Mary Barksdale, Pamela Van Bogart-Dufek, Cary Leach, Jani Scheepstra, Serhat Ozkacak, Massimilliano Venturi, Ibriham Aldesoki, Ricky Peterson, James Tichota, Joan Smith, Sarah J. Davis, Romy Stitch, Jen Springer Rupert, Felipe De La Riva, Amy Marie, Michael Tierno, Teresa Lautrup, Charlie Jeff Whitley, Dwight Brooks, Michael Joe Demko, Richard Perry, Jonathan Roberts, Rick Bock, Uxmal Reyes, Kelley Lynn Davis Hankins, Nick Roach, Patrick Matthew, Sophie Kirby, Joy Elyse Nadel, Janine Fredenberg-Toth, Brenda Peters, Julia May, Laura Helena Denton, Melissa Clark-Pensiero, Tari Elsenar, Brenda Dawson, Janelle Jubainville-Connell, April Krass, Aiden RC, Inez Walker, Robert Rocha, Katie Clark, Michelle Savage Clement, Inez Walker, Emily Klaras, James Farmer, Mickie Kuchinski Mace, Teri Sayble Killin, Swaroop Dogra, Victoria Gerber, Erika Sanchez, Heather Grindstaff, Shashawnee Lisenbee, Jitendra Maloo, Mickie Foris, Anne Schmidt Francisco, Sarah Noelle Hammond, Cleveland Wheeler, Savannah Chandler, and Sultan Zafar, Xev Setter, Corrine Brandel-Valencia, Tony Cotto, Donnie Ferguson, Vincente Patino Fernandez, Cleveland Wheeler, Antoinette Ricardo, Clara Jimenez, Morena, Nancy Kolovitz, Darlene Been Watkins, Mike Lynn, Andrea Ragsdale, Marion Adler Young, David Todd, Melissa Gs, Sheila Castleberg Kalish, Elizabeth Wicander, Britt Wise, Debra Pierce Bellare, Nicole Miner Alford, Rachel Schreiberman, Ronald Willams, Jeff Dirk Donavan, John Salazar, Kayla Lee, Tysons Mammy, Ashely Coomer, Marla Sexton, Sara Riquelme, Nancy Kolovitz, Dianna Brock Carter, Stephanie Holmes, Clara Jimenez Moreno, Koen Suidgeest, Elizabeth Berner, Antoinette Ricardo, Dianna Brock Carter,

Stephanie Holmes, Dynesha Briley, Fabienne Hyden, Jitendra Maloo, America Proctor, Bianca Ballwanz, Katie Dryden, Sara Larken, Lucky Ollie, JD Vehorn, Wendy Spahn, Kaylin Nickerson, Jodi Indiveri Pharis, and Joe Hecht, Elizabeth Theresa, and Denise Ford.

Also, watch for the cartoon "Little Billy" written by Chance Raspberry, the Simpsons' Lead Animator!

PROLOGUE

"I'm coldddd…!" Jani shivers a scream.

"You were hot a minute ago." I keep calm. Jani is thirteen now. She knows better than to act this way, especially inside a restaurant. We're at the Olive Garden in Valencia, the quiet town twenty minutes north of Los Angeles where we live. It is even called "Awesome Town."

There aren't many restaurants our family can go to because Jani is a vegetarian and won't eat just "anywhere." Bodhi is an omnivore but needs a bright atmosphere because he's afraid of the dark. Sometimes, like today, even that is not enough. "I wanna take my eyes out," Bodhi gets up from his chair and hides himself inside my chest. "But if I take my eyes out then there'll be blood." He looks up at me.

"Yes, Bodhi. So don't do it," I respond rationally to Bodhi's bizarre question, which I believe to be a symptom of schizophrenia. *I wish the behaviorist would get here.* "We just ordered our food and drinks are on the way."

"I'm soooooo cold," Jani continues to whine.

"You should always bring a jacket." I keep my patience in check.

"I'll chew!" As long as I can remember, Jani has chewed on long sleeves and jacket cuffs, so I just mutter a sigh.

"If you take your eyes out…then there will be blood," Bodhi repeats like he's reading a sentence from a children's horror encyclopedia. I remember his blanket in the car. *I curse myself for not remembering this simple solution sooner.*

"Yes, Bodhi," I say, secretly hoping this may be a career path to becoming an ophthalmologist before returning my attention to Jani. "Why don't you go out to the car and get Bodhi's blanket?" The last time we were in a restaurant it worked perfectly. We used the blanket to block out whatever Bodhi was seeing, then floated it across the table to keep Jani warm. Valencia is always warm, hot, or broiling, not cold. Even in the wintertime, cold is rare, which is why every restaurant is air-conditioned and we keep a blanket in the car.

"No! I'm not going!" Jani screams.

"Then you'll just have to be cold." I mimic her obstinacy. UCLA told us that as she grew up we'd have the same problems other parents have with their teenagers on top of the mental illness.

"Mommy!" Bodhi clutches me, seemingly scared. I tuck him under my arm as the smiling waitress brings our drink orders on a wooden server tray.

Jani reaches out to get her drink, but stops, appearing to control herself. "I'm SOOOOOO COOOOLDD!"

"Jani! We're *not* staying if you're going to keep screaming." She hiccups a fake cry, taking one of the drinks from the waitress's hand, but before she can set it down on the table...it's too late. In a flash, Bodhi grabs my large Diet Coke and flings it into the air while time and motion stand still. Droplets of Diet Coke sprinkle high above the crowd eating before hitting the back of a guy's chair, making him jerk his shoulder around as the glass shatters into small pieces on the floor.

A stunned chorus of "OH's!" echo around us. If only I hadn't been arguing with Jani? If only our 23-year-old behaviorist, Alysha, had arrived earlier? If only...? "It's okay," the waitress says nervously, like this happens all the time.

"Thank you, but we're leaving, *now*," I say, pointedly at Jani, spotting Alysha, out-of-breath as she rushes through a maze of tables to reach Bodhi. He's crying, just as surprised by his actions as the rest of us are.

"I threw the Diet Coke?!?" He questions me, a look of horror on his face.

"Yes, you threw the Diet Coke and now we're going home."

"No!" Jani says adamantly before whimpering "Why?" as though none of this registered with her either.

"Because you're not behaving and you don't *deserve* to go out to a restaurant! We'll try again another time." *Damn. I really want that cheese ravioli.* But I have to make an impression on her. Jani is almost fourteen and has to learn how to act in a restaurant. As for Bodhi, even after all we've been through, he's still not on the right medication. I take one last look around at the crowd. Surprisingly, they've all gone back to eating as though nothing happened, but the evidence glitters in the glass shards on the floor in front of us.

PART ONE

CHAPTER 1

FIRST COMES LOVE,
THEN COMES MARRIAGE

April 24th, 1999

Los Angeles, "The City of Angels," never sleeps. Most down-town areas are well-lit, offering a safe and peaceful glow. I brake at the stoplight. It's just after 3 am and I just got off work reporting the news and traffic for Doug Stephan's syndicated radio show. To-night was mostly Columbine updates. How could the parents NOT know their sons were building bombs in the garage and planning to blow up their school in Colorado, killing other kids...?

I just don't get it.

The stoplight is taking a long time to turn green and there aren't any cars behind me. I'm not in a hurry, but I would like to get home and just sleep next to Michael. We've been engaged for two years and we're going to get married next year.

When I look to my right, a tall thin man with solidly white hair slowly steps off the street corner. He is using a thick braided rope as a leash for his dog. As he walks through the crosswalk, I can see the dog's ribcage. He must be homeless but he's neatly dressed in light blue denim. I can't look away. I always give to homeless people when I have the money, especially when they have dogs. *They're walking in my path for a reason.*

I roll my down my car window as the light turns green, and call out to him. "Sir, do you need any money?" He stops in his tracks and we make eye contact. His bright blue eyes match his denim jacket. "Can you feed your dog?" I'm lucky there aren't any cars behind me. In fact, there aren't any cars anywhere close.

"I can barely feed myself," he saunters up to my open window, peeking inside my car, then straightening back up. "I have cancer," he says matter-of-factly. I look down at his dog, then back up at the stoplight turning from yellow to red. "I found her, barking, tied up to a tree. I think the owner just left her there," he shrugs. "So, I cut off the rope with my knife."

"What's her name?" I ask him.

"I call her Ronin." He lets down his guard.

I look down at Ronin, her expressive brown eyes speaking to mine. I put my hand down in front of her nose and she licks me, her tongue, scratchy and sweet. "Do you want me to take her?" The words fly out of my mouth, seizing me in the moment.

"Would you?" His eyes beg.

I stare up at the stoplight to remind myself that I'm really here and not locked inside some sort of dream state. The light is green. I look around again. Surely, someone should be honking at me by now, forcing me to leave in a hurry. Amazingly for Los Angeles, no one is here. I think about where Michael and I live. It's just the two of us in a two-bedroom apartment near Burbank that allows big dogs. Besides, with her gray-white muzzle, she's probably about ten years old.

I pet her soft auburn fur. Her body is so thin I can feel her rib cage popping out of her. She'll probably just lay around the place, but we'll be able to keep her comfortable.

"Yes. I can take her," I answer firmly. Then, without another thought, I get out of my car and walk around to the back door of the passenger's side and open it. She's so tired from walking that after stepping into my car she just drops to the floor of the back seat, curling her body into a tight ball of dog. The man reaches into his pocket and pulls out a switchblade. He flicks it open and I just stand there, knowing I'm okay, even though I probably should NOT feel okay about any of this. He cuts the rope from her neck and closes his blade, shoving it back into his pocket. "God bless you."

"God bless you, too" I smile, knowing in my heart that I am doing the right thing. I search my purse for anything to give him. I find four one-dollar bills and hand them over. "This is all I have."

"Thank you," he says, more kind than desperate.

"By the way, do you how old is she?"

"Mmm?" He questions the air, "I think she was born around Thanksgiving last year."

"Oh," I blink my doubt and wave good-bye. This man must be crazy. This dog is not that young, but it doesn't matter. He nods, graciously, sliding his hands into his jean pockets as he looks anxiously from side to side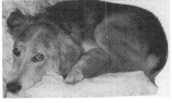

Honey taking one for the team.

to see if anyone is behind him. Then he quickens his pace and steps onto the opposite side of the street, almost like he'd expected to be alone when he got there.

This time, when the light turns green, I make my left turn toward the freeway. I try catching a last glance of him, but he's already disappeared into the night. I look over my shoulder. "Don't worry, honey, I'm going to bring you home. We'll take care of you." That's it! "Honey! What a great name! And it fits you because you're so sweet and honey-colored."

It's a quiet drive home. I hope Michael will be okay with me bringing Honey home. I can't imagine he wouldn't want to keep her as much as I do. After all, it won't be long before we're married and this is good practice for a baby.

*　　*　　*

Michael is my first real relationship. We met a few years earlier when I was working as a board operator for KFI AM 640. Back then, Rush Limbaugh and Dr. Laura were at the height of their careers and the catch phrase was "More Stimulating Talk Radio." I pressed lots of buttons to keep the station alive, thinking of myself as an airline pilot with all these controls in front of me. One wrong move and that's it…dead air.

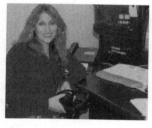

When I replay the previous broadcasts, I make sure never to autopilot. Instead, I practice hosting my own talk show with Dave the Engineer and "Old Mike," the 27-year-old board operator I'm "in love with." The problem is that he's married. Not that

Susan working night shift. he didn't offer and not that I never wanted to accept his offer, but after 25 years of saving myself for "The One," the last thing I'm about to do is lose my virginity with a married man.

Just like in any other job, we grow closer during downtime. In our case, the light is dim, mimicking a VIP room at a nightclub, minus the drugs and alcohol. "I want to get married, but only to a man who truly loves me," I tell them

"You're lucky you're *not* married." Dave leans back in his chair, apathetically. He is in his 40s, struggling with his own marriage.

"But I want to be. I just need to find the right guy."

"Oh," he gives me a crooked smile, closing his eyes, picturing some sort of personal hell. "Juuusst…wait…until the bags come…"

"Everyone has baggage."

"Yes, but her bags just keep coming," he nods to himself. "No, actually, they're *suitcases*. She did things in her past that I had no idea about." Dave is emphatic, shaking his head.

"That's why I'm taking my time."

"Look, guys give love to get sex," Dave says as if it's written in stone, "And girls…they give sex, to get love."

"Then how do you know if it's true love?"

"You don't," he says flatly. I shake my head. This is so hard to believe. Here I am, waiting for "The One," and Dave is telling me there is no "One."

Old Mike, comes out of the editing studio and my heart jumps. I can't control it. "So, what do you think?" I ask him flirtatiously as Dr. Laura, famous for her book *Ten Stupid Things Women Do to Mess Up Their Lives*, airs in the background.

"Dave's right," he says.

"So, does every husband cheat on his wife then?"

"It's not just men," Old Mike squint-eyes me. "It's women too." He and Dave exchange all-knowing grins.

Oh, thank God! My New Michael is walking in. He's the reason I call Mike "Old Mike." Michael and I have been getting really close lately. The day we met he said I was cute and I returned the compliment. I add him to our conversation. "Do you believe in true love…that a man and woman can be faithful to each other?"

"Sure," he says, adding flippantly, "Whales mate for life." His blue eyes are so serious, intelligent. Old Mike lets out a spontaneous laugh and Dave rolls his eyes.

But they don't know. My New Michael is way beyond these guys. I just learned something new so I make sure to educate them. "See…whales mate for life."

Old Mike is clearly frustrated, as he checks out this New Michael from head to toe. "At least I'm honest about it."

My heart doesn't flutter for Michael like it does for Old Mike, but he is cute and walks with a confident swagger. His black boots add to the lanky stature I love. "If you can envision it," he tells me over the phone one night, "then it's already happened."

"WOW!" I take the time to process this thought. It's like I'm learning something new every day and I absolutely *love* the way he thinks! It's like he takes my thoughts and magnifies them. The only problem is that I'm almost twenty-six with my eyes on marriage and a family; Michael is only twenty. But he's amazing! He answers every question I ask immediately with a bonus air of sophistication and confidence other guys just don't have. He seems older than his years.

We both want to be writers. As we start seeing each other every day, we find out that we have so much more in common. This is the first time I don't have to explain myself to someone. He doesn't just immediately 'get' my ideas. Instead of balking at them, he takes them even further.

When he asks me to go on a writing venture to Las Vegas with him, I'm a little hesitant. The thought of how much fun would it be to work and play at the same time convinces me. This is the first of many trips we take to Vegas to flesh out our movie-making ideas. He drives and I take notes, keeping a tape recorder at my side.

Besides, what am I waiting for? Maybe Old Mike prepared me for this. I'm willing to take this next step because New Michael is, among other things, single. I make him get two rooms, but we never use the second one. I technically remain a virgin for another year, but we get a lot closer than I ever imagined. I'd never had this much fun before in my life!

*   *   *

As soon as I finish the drive home from downtown, I wake up Michael and tell him everything. He helps me get Honey out of the backseat and carry her into our apartment. "We've got to get her to a vet," he says. I love the way Michael just takes over when I need him. He searches the Internet and finds a 24-hour vet just fifteen minutes away. They tell us the homeless man was right. Honey is a puppy! She is a Golden Retriever/Aussie Shepherd mix. Honey bonds to me immediately and she's very social, at least when it comes to dog parks and daycare.

We learned early on not to take her on road trips. When we went to the Grand Canyons, she waited a full twenty hours to do her business and then she just peed. As we drove to Flagstaff, she yelped and five minutes later, she finally pooped–all over the car.

Luckily, we found a pet store that cleaned her up while Michael paid $100 to get the car cleaned. After that, we put her in boarding at the vet when we traveled.

Honey was great with the vet and very social in doggie daycare, but she was extremely territorial at home. It got to the point that she nipped at our friends and family if they got too close. Her bark was worse than her bite, but when people got scared, it made her behavior worse. We stopped inviting people inside our home for the next few years.

April 14th, 2000

Michael and I elope to Vegas. Michael wanted to forego alcohol at our wedding and I agreed with him because, really, what did I care? I've never liked alcohol and it was our wedding. Unfortunately, this was such a big issue with my family that they canceled our wedding. Happily, this left us free to wed in the place we felt most comfortable: The Monte Carlo in Las Vegas. Besides, I just want to get our life started and, most importantly, I want a baby.

*   *   *

Michael and I are still writing but when we get to a certain point, we just can't make any more progress on our screenplays. It's time for a new plan, so I support Michael going back to school to get his BA in English. As his new life begins, he seems like a kid enjoying his newfound freedom and I become more of a mother-figure to him. On November 19th, 2001, he really hits a chord. "I thought you were going to be with me tonight." He already knows from my expression that I am upset with him.

"I won't be gone all night. It's just that Rodrigo and I need to finish our writing project."

"But you didn't tell me you were going to do this?"

"Huh," he sighs.

"And you never told me where you're going?"

"Rodrigo can't get off from work tonight so I have to go where he works."

"Where's that?"

"Some nightclub."

"WHAT?! We made a deal, remember? No nightclubs! Why can't you just go to a coffee shop? You're the one who didn't want any alcohol at our wedding. Remember? That's why it was canceled and we went to Vegas?"

"Yes, but Rodrigo has to work."

"He works at a nightclub?" I shake my head at him, then gulp my fear. "So, how's he going to have time to write with you?"

"He's the bartender."

"He's the BARTENDER?! That's even WORSE! You're going to be sitting at a bar while Rodrigo's working and other girls are going to be drinking around you."

Michael sighs. "It's not like that...."

"Okay," I soften, my eyes misty, thinking about what is really happening here. He kisses me and I know his resolve is weakening. *I've got him!* As we keep kissing, there's a knock at the door. I know its Rodrigo.

"Uh...hold on," he calls out to the door.

"Please," I turn on my inner Playboy Bunny, "Don't go."

He strolls over to the door, cracking it open, then looking back at me. "Uh, I'm gonna have to cancel tonight," he lowers his head.

"Are you sure?" I walk closer to the door, looking over Michael's shoulder, just enough for Rodrigo to know the reason why. "Okay, man," he seems to get the picture. "I'll catch you later."

Michael closes the door and turns back to me. I smile as we race into the bedroom. It isn't the first time we skipped using birth control, but I tell him that he doesn't need it since I never get pregnant. And I am right... until tonight.

CHAPTER 2

THEN COMES BABY IN A BABY CARRIAGE

January 10th, 2002

"You're going to have to get rid of her." Both our families have the same response when we announce our pregnancy.

"We can't do that?!" I look to Michael.

"We're not going to," he stands strong. "Honey will be *fine* with the baby."

"Maybe you should just get a doll that cries so she can get used to the noise." We do this, but Honey just cocks her head to both sides, her ears perking up. Otherwise, she doesn't know what to make of it. There's an on-off switch on the back of the doll, but it affects us more than it does Honey, so we prefer to keep the switch off as much as possible.

*　　　*　　　*

January 10th, 2002 is our very first ultrasound.

"Stop giggling. We can't see the image on the screen." Michael has the advantage of seeing everything in real time. I try to hold still so the screen will stop scrambling and let the image come into focus.

"I can't help it." Tears sprinkle over my cheeks. "I still can't be-lieve I'm pregnant."

"Well, you are," Michael takes a closer look. "And there's our baby," he points. "It looks like all the limbs are already formed."

"That's interesting. Your baby is really...out there," Dr. Matz takes a closer look at the image as she wiggles the wand to get a bet-ter view. "I don't usually get a full picture like this. Your baby is right in front of the camera."

"Then our baby is definitely going to be a Leo."

Dr. Matz smiles. "Yep, your due date is August 11th." She puts the wand away and hands me my first image of my first baby. I can't seem to stop laughing and crying at the same time. Before we leave, a friendly nurse loads me up with sample vitamins.

*　　　*　　　*

I snuggle in close to Michael as we watch Olympic figure skat-ing. We've already picked out our baby names: January or Derrick. "You know, if we do have a girl, maybe she'll be an ice skater and we can write a book about her. We'll call it *January on Ice*." I smile.

"I still think we're having a boy."

"According to the Chinese Calendar...."

"I know, I know," he interrupts, mocking me.

On March 20th, 2002, we get the big ultrasound. I'm so giddy right now, I can't hold back. "According to the Chinese Calendar," I tell the lady tech, "I'm having a girl."

"So, you both want to know what the gender is then?" Her eyes dart back and forth at us.

"YES!" I scream.

"Yeah," Michael also agrees. We're finally going to find out if I'm having a boy or a girl!

"You know, the lady starts spreading the cool gel on my stom-ach, "As long as I've been here, I'd say that about 85% of the time, the Chinese Calendar has been right."

"See," I tell Michael who's rooting for a son. I'm clenching my teeth, praying. I've always wanted a daughter since as long as I could remember. She uses the white ultrasound Doppler to get a picture. For me, this time when the image comes onto the screen, like we're watching a movie, is the best part about being pregnant. Her finger stops for a moment to click a button and the photo is taken. "Is everything okay?" I ask.

"Everything looks good," she nods, eyeing the computer in front of her. "See, there's the brain flow," she points to the thick blue and red lines moving horizontally across the screen.

"Whew." I breathe a sigh of relief, carefully watching her expressions.

"So, what is that?" I ask, unable to figure out the new picture.

"Hold on…" She puts her Doppler on another part of my stomach. "I'm going to say that I'm 95 percent sure. It's a…girl!"

My mouth is stuck in the "AW" position and I can't get it to close. Then, I burst out with laughing tears. *God answered my prayers! He's giving me a daughter!*

"Wait," Michael walks closer to the screen. "You mean that's not a penis?"

"Nope," the lady tech says. "Right here," she moves the Doppler for a closer view. "Those are her legs, wide open. That's the labia." She nods over to Michael, then me. "Make that 99 percent." She moves out for a wide shot and we see a detailed side view of Jani.

"Look, she's coughing in there," I point.

"And her hands. It's like she's waving at us," Michael tears up and I don't think I'll ever get the grin off my face as the tech takes some more close-up pictures.

"She's beautiful, just like I thought she'd be. And, she looks like you," I say to Michael.

"Yeah. She does," he starts to tear up again.

*   *   *

In May, the tension rises as our due date nears. "Your daughter's a brat," Dr. Matz grimaces, her stethoscope searching out Jani's heartbeat.

"Well, she is going to be a Leo," I emphasize, knowing Dr. Matz is also and how particular she is about *everything*. Since I was in high school, I've always wanted a Leo daughter because all my Leo friends had boundless energy that I didn't. They got straight A's, were in drama, on the cheerleading squad, and ALWAYS popular.

"Yeah, well, I'm a Leo too and I'm a brat," Dr. Matz grimaces, getting more frustrated, circling around me.

"What's wrong?" Now, I'm getting nervous.

"I can't find her heartbeat."

"What?!" I look up at Michael, my shoulders tensing up.

"No, it's not that," Dr. Matz shakes her head. I know she's there. She just won't stop moving."

"Ohhh," my shoulders fall in relief. "Well, she hardly ever sleeps. I know because when I work the overnight shift, she's up and then when I go to sleep in the day, I can still feel her moving around."

"Ahhh," Dr. Matz rests her stethoscope on my stomach, like a Lioness who caught her cub while I look up at Michael as he rubs my stomach reassuringly.

*   *   *

It's Memorial Day and my parents have come to visit for the weekend. Right now we're stuck in holiday traffic, making our way north to Santa Barbara on the 101. I've always got my hand on my stomach these days so I know when Jani is sleeping, which isn't often or long. That's why the last two hours have me on edge. She's never that quiet in there. "Jani's not moving?!"

"She's probably sleeping," my mom says dismissively.

"No, you don't understand. She never sleeps like this! She just takes short naps," I tell her as scary scenarios run through my head.

"She has to sleep sometime. How long has it been?"

"Two hours."

"That's nothing." My mom waves me off. "She'll wake up at

some point. Remember, you're getting closer to delivery."

"I'm just paranoid." For the first time, but not the last, I work to convince myself that what we're experiencing is normal.

"It will be okay."

*   *   *

I'm still on edge as we stroll Santa Barbara's side streets full of antique stores and craft shops. My parents look at souvenirs while Michael tries to find something special for his new daughter. I'm too preoccupied with what is going on with January inside me to relax.

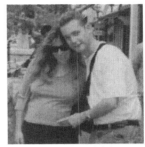

"I'm in the mood for a good steak. Let's stop here," Michael says when we stumble on Chuck's Steak House. As we sit around *Susan, Michael, and Jani (in utero) in Santa Barbara.*

the table preparing to order, January finally moves! I'm relieved enough to eat my chicken dinner in peace. After the waiter brings our drinks, I'm so relaxed that I take my mom's criticisms easily.

"How do you think she's going to like her name?" my mom starts out.

"I like the name," my dad nods. "I remember when Susan first heard it in that old movie we were watching, '*Once is Not Enough*'."

"Yeah, I like it too," Michael says.

"Both Michael and Dad were born in January. Also, it's the perfect name for a model. And what if she is? I can tell she has Michael's body so she'll probably be tall and thin."

My mom shakes her head. "Well, I don't like it."

"She can always be called Jani or even Jan if she wants to."

"Just don't leave Honey around the baby alone," my dad warns.

"We're not planning to, but Honey will be fine," Michael says, adamantly. We are both so sick of hearing this.

Years later, we find out that Jani had a minor stroke, probably in utero. The possibility that Jani had a stroke while we strolled around

Santa Barbara haunts me. What happened to Jani that day? We will never know.

*   *   *

Before I go on maternity leave, my friend Judy suggests that right after Jani is born, we take a piece of her baby clothes and let Honey smell it before they meet. After we're home a couple days, Michael picks Honey up from boarding. He has a piece of clothing Jani's spit-up is already on. Before walking in, I see him through the door, letting her sniff it.

We're so confident that she won't hurt Jani that I have Michael videotape their first encounter so we can show the world. I sit cross-legged our dark green futon while Michael leads Honey into the liv-

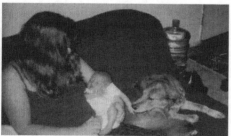

ing room and starts filming. We have faith in our Honey. Slowly, Honey walks over to me holding Jani in my arms, sniffs her head, then walks quietly over to the corner of our living room. No barking,

Photographic proof that Honey was fine with Jani.

no lunging, no nothing. It's like she instinctively knows that Jani is part of our pack. I thank God for Honey. Who knew that *our pet* would be our guiding light for what was to come?

*   *   *

Just like in the womb, Jani rarely sleeps, catnapping 20 to 30 minutes around the clock, getting 4 to 5 hours of sleep in a 24-hour period. Michael and I are on our own to keep her entertained all day so that she will give us the two to three hours that most parents of newborns complain about. Oh, sure we'd heard the stories of other babies sleeping for twelve, sixteen, even twenty hours straight, but we didn't believe them.

Everyone around us keeps saying to get her into a routine. We do, but our routine is different. Unlike everyone else, we have to stimulate her all day, every day, to get that full eight hours at night. Finding a mom's group–several actually–is a big help for me. When Jani finishes a playdate with one toddler, it is on to the next friend. Michael and I split it 50/50. Each of us has a break. We live off of my part-time radio shifts and Michael's student loans.

Over the next few years, Michael graduates from Cal State Northridge with a BA in English and immediately continues on toward an MA so he can teach at the college level and earn more money. This works out well for Jani because she and Michael have such a strong bond. He constantly teaches her at a level that is beyond me.

*　　*　　*

When it's my turn to care for Jani all day, we go to the Burbank Mall where there's this small toy store that lures other mothers and their babies because the back is a play area with cushioned blue mats, baby toys, plastic climbing structures, and most importantly, a gate. Moms can sit and rest, knowing their babies are safely entertained. Having other moms to talk to is like Heaven. The best part is that for just five dollars I can come and go throughout the day.

Today, I take Jani out for some fresh air along the sidewalk on San Fernando Blvd. This is where I meet Lynn. She's coming out of the bookstore and *she has a stroller! Yay!* And this stroller carries twin girls about Jani's age. *Friends!!!* I immediately stop to talk to her. After all, when you're a new mom, you're automatically in the "New Mom's Club." No need to fill out any membership form.

"Hi," I say, seeing the weary look on her face that is so familiar to me when I look in the mirror.

"Hi," she smiles back.

"How old are they?" I ask.

"Nine months."

"How old is she?" Lynn asks.

"Six months," I tell her, then add, "Do you know about Sweet Little Faces? It's a play area for babies in the mall..."

"Where is it?"

She's interested! "It's right by Sears on the 3rd floor."

"I'll have to check that out," she says, appreciatively.

"I'll be going back there in a bit. I'm just getting some coffee now."

"Okay, well, maybe we'll see you there."

We say our good-byes and about two hours later I see her walk in with her stroller, looking over the area like it's a heaven she never knew existed. I wave at her excitedly and she pays the small fee for each of them. Then she joins me and we relax and talk for hours. This is the beginning of a friendship that lasts to this day.

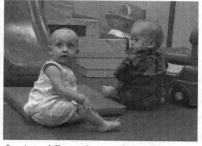

A couple months later, I meet Bethanne and her fifteen-month-old son, Brandon. My group grows to include Andrea, her son Lee, Cathy, and Eli.

We meet on most weekdays for nearly two years, from the time

Jani and Brandon at Sweet Little Faces.

Jani is almost one until the other kids start preschool. We start to lose touch with Lee when his parent's divorce. Eli has some problems with aggression and pushing, so we mostly call them for play-dates at the zoo and other flat places.

These moms see it all from the beginning. They know there is more going on than Jani being a spoiled brat. These moms are my friends and support system, and their kids are Jani's friends. They are the first ones to suggest we seek medical help for her. Later, when other people only see an angry, beaten-down Michael, they still remember when Michael was at his best with Jani.

*   *   *

While Michael is going to school at Northridge, we move to a new, cheaper apartment closer to there. Now, Michael's commute is shorter, but mine is longer. We're further away from Jani's friends but we think it's worth it, until we realize the water in our new apartment goes out every few months. We would move back to Burbank, but Honey is 43 pounds and no apartments take a dog over 40 pounds. We try putting her on a diet, but it just doesn't work. Plus, Honey would never pass any dog interview.

We are lucky and find an even more beautiful apartment complex in Valencia that is cheaper and takes big dogs. Honey doesn't even need to do a doggy interview because that she is a golden retriever, Australian shepherd mix. Even though we're now a half-hour away from my Moms' group, there is a luxurious pool and my friends love to visit.

CHAPTER 3

SEVERELY GIFTED

Summer 2006

"They don't get my imagination," Jani complains as Lynn and her four-year-old twins, Elizabeth and Corrine, drive through the gate to our apartment complex. With the summer heat, we're all more than ready to go swimming. The problem is that Jani's imaginary friends consume so much of her time that she's isolating herself from the real friends she's grown up with since she was a baby, including Elizabeth and Corinne.

"They're identical twins, Jani. They have their own special language, but Lynn's bringing another girl for you to meet. Maybe she'll get your imagination?"

"Is that the new girl?" Jani points to a white SUV following Lynn's Caravan.

"I think so." Jani smiles as a bubbly, brown-haired girl waves anxiously out the window. Her mom stops the car to park. *Maybe, just maybe, she'll get Jani's imagination.*

"Hi, I'm Lily," the little girl pops out of her Mom's car dressed in pink sandals and an Ariel princess bathing suit.

"I'm Blue-Eyed Tree Frog," Jani responds.

"Jani has a big imagination," I automatically shift into explanation-mode. "She likes to change her name."

"Lily loves to pretend too," Lily's mom smiles warmly as we take the girls to the pool to find shade under the wine-colored cabanas. Elizabeth and Corrine toss their swim toys into the pool while Jani stands by me.

"Girls, you need sunblock!" Lynn calls over to her daughters as they're about to step into the water with Lily following suit.

"You too, Lily!" her mom echoes.

"400 is here," Jani whispers in my ear as I'm applying her sunscreen. "She says she's going to splatter mango juice on the twins."

"Well as long as she doesn't do it," I smile at my creative daughter, knowing full well that there isn't even mango juice around for her imaginary cat to throw.

"Jani!" Lily calls out to her, ready to play after the twins have already jumped into the pool.

"I'm NOT Jani! I'm Wednesday!"

Uh-oh. "Jani, Lily and the girls are your guests. You have to be nice!"

"I thought she was Blue-Eyed Tree Frog," Lynn turns to me as Lily's mom watches.

"She's been switching names lately, several times a day now, and it's getting annoying." Lynn nods. "Jani's a little different than most kids," I tell Lily's mom.

"She's 'unique'," Lynn corrects me with a smile.

"I'm NOT Jani!"

"Then just pick a name and go with it!" I call over to her.

"I'm Ariel the Mermaid," Lily splashes, playfully, in the pool.

I turn back to the moms. "I figure that people have nicknames so she can have one too, but she needs to choose one. Otherwise, kids are going to get confused."

Lily jumps out of the pool. "Come on Wednesday," she waves

Jani over to the hot tub and Jani happily follows, with the twins trailing them. "Who are you?" Lily asks Corrine.

"Sll-ee-pp—ing Beauty," Corrine stammers, looking down at her swimsuit.

"Me...tt-oo." Elizabeth looks over at her sister for silent confirmation.

"My girls are in Speech Therapy. They have a stuttering problem we're trying to fix before kindergarten," Lynn explains.

"I think they're all doing great," Lily's mom says. "They're playing so nicely together."

"That reminds me, Susan. I meant to tell you, I met a woman whose son has Asperger's. He's nine now and she wishes she'd gotten him diagnosed earlier because the longer you wait, the harder it becomes."

"We're going to get her tested this fall," I answer Lynn's unasked question, "Along with her IQ. We know she's brilliant." I look over at Jani, who's now out of the hot tub and crawling under the coffee table near the fireplace. "Jani, please go back to the hot tub with the other girls."

"I'm playing with 400!"

"Who's 400?" Lily's mom asks.

"It's her imaginary cat friend."

"Oh," Lily's mom chuckles.

"Why don't you just bring 400 over to play with your real friends," I get off the chaise lounge.

"She doesn't like them."

Shit. I cringe.

"Girls, can you go back to the pool and show January your new swim toys?" Lynn asks her twins.

"I'M NOT JANUARY!"

"I mean Blue-Eyed Tree Frog," Lynn quickly corrects herself.

"IT'S WEDNESDAY!" Jani screams.

"Jani!" I'm growing more impatient. "You're not going to have friends if you don't pick a name and just GO WITH IT!"

"But I'm not Jani."

"Lily, why don't you go over to where Wednesday's playing?" Lily's mom suggests.

"Okay," Lily complies. Wow, what an easy child. Even Lynn's twins aren't this agreeable. Soon, all the girls are gathered around Jani and crawling around on the furniture by the fireplace.

"I'm sorry," I apologize again. "I'm trying to get Jani to socialize better."

"I'm doing the same with my girls too," Lynn admits. "They usually just play with each other."

"Lily's an only child and I'm too old to have any more, so she knows she has to make friends."

We relax and snack on Teddy Grahams and bottled water as the girls play, but soon the twins are off by themselves again, on the other side of the pool. At least Jani and Lily are playing together. What a relief. "Are you hungry for a snack, Lily?" Her mom asks.

"No. I'm playing in Calalini."

"Calalini?" Lily's mom asks me, between snacking.

"It's where 400 lives," I explain.

"I've got to get Lily into acting classes before we leave," Lily's mom says. "She loves pretending."

"Before you leave?" I ask, my heart sinking.

"Yeah, we're moving to Colorado in the fall." My jaw drops.

"I'm going to miss them too," Lynn says but she's not half as distraught as I am. I know it's not easy raising twin girls but at least they each have a built-in playmate. Jani only has imaginary friends.

*   *   *

Jani's pediatrician refers us to an educational psychologist, Heidi Yellen. Michael and I are both relieved when Heidi talks to her for a while and says, "No, she doesn't have Asperger's, she's way too engaging. I want to give her an IQ test." By this point, Jani has tons of imaginary friends, but she manages to keep them outside while she takes the test, allowing her to score an amazing 146 on the SB5 at just four years and two months old. (The Stanford-Binet Intelligence Scales, Fifth Edition is the most recent version of this commonly used IQ assessment tool; scores max out around 145, which is significantly lower than on older versions of the test.)

"She broke the test. You need to get her into a gifted school, immediately." She gives us a moment to digest this as we sit on her couch like befuddled students. "This didn't happen by accident."

"But I've already checked them out and they have interviews. She'll scream if she's called January and besides that, she won't potty train. Well, technically her pediatrician says that she actually is potty-trained because she doesn't have accidents in the day or night. She just uses her pull-ups as her potty. But she has to use the toilet to go to school."

Most of her oldest friends, including the twins and Brandon, have been in preschool for years. Lee is even in kindergarten, but since we can't get Jani to use the toilet, our never-ending task of keeping her stimulated on our own continues. Of course, Dr. Yellen tells us to potty-train her immediately, as if we weren't already trying everything we could think of.

*   *   *

Christmas week 2006, Michael is off from teaching. There is no better time than the present. *Please, God, give us this one gift.* Unlike other children, Jani cannot be bribed with candy, toys, or other objects. The one thing she *needs* is to go out every single day, in sickness and in health. Since she was two and a half months old, we have accommodated her. Our choice was to listen to constant screaming or bring her out and the screaming stopped, immediately.

I make new rules. "You can use your pull-ups as the potty like you've been doing, but you can't leave home until you pee in the potty. Daddy and I can leave, one at a time, but until you choose to cooperate, you have to stay at home."

Jani is old enough now that she knows the rules and agrees, but after three days at home, we're both losing hope. This is unbeliev able. I suppose the good news is that now we know that we can stay home for a day, or two, even three! She can watch television, videos, play with her toys, even work on the computer. This is great news for when either of us is sick.

I remember telling Michael when she was a baby that by the time she's five we would be able to reason with her. Reaching this goal post has kept us going for all these years. Michael remains the pessimist. "It's not working." I know he's right, but I can't give up. Michael doesn't understand that when he's ready to "give up," it makes me more determined to prove him wrong.

He holds the door open, head hanging low as he leads Honey out. "How long are you going to be gone?"

"About twenty minutes," he says. I know it will really be closer to forty minutes.

"You know what?"

"Yeah?" he questions my question.

"I'm going to have her potty-trained by the time you get back."

"Huh," he muffles a laugh and walks out the door, leaving me watching Jani glued to the TV. It took years before she could even do that.

*　　*　　*

I practice the deep breathing techniques that my Zen Friend, Michi, has been teaching me for years. Michi and I met when Michael worked with her husband at Mailboxes Etc. in Burbank. Their daughter, Grace, was just two at the time. We lost touch for a while when Michael started school at Northridge, but we reconnected at the Barnes & Noble in Valencia when Grace was eight and Jani was just three and a half.

Unlike most people, Grace and Michi love Jani's imagination. Grace works as a child actress, so Michi is homeschooling her. We see them a lot and practice what Grace calls "FunZen." FunZen uses tools from Michi's book *Mental Fitness* to make meditation techniques kid-friendly.

*   *   *

It's time. Jani is squiggling around. She needs to use the potty. She'll pick up a pull-up I've carefully laid out for her, per our agreement. I didn't want to take them away entirely because I thought that just staying home would get her past this irrational fear but I was clearly wrong.

I'm keeping a close eye on the very last training pants. It can't be long now. Another few minutes go by while I wait on the edge of my seat. Then it happens. Jani saunters over to where her pull-up is beside the wall. She's ready to put it on, pee, or poop, then promptly throw it away in the trash, but she doesn't get there in time. In a flash, I race over, snagging the training pants as she's about to grab it. I got it! *Now what do I do?!*

"Unnh," she whimpers, reaching for the training pants I hold high over my head.

"No. You need to use the potty. I know you have to go. *You* know you have to go. Just do it now and get it over with!"

"I want that pull-up," her voice regains strength, only this time, she's dead serious, but I'm way taller than she is so I keep my arm steady, high above me, as she reaches for it. Her whimper turns to an angry cry. "Give me that pull-up!"

"No!" She jumps up and I'm actually getting a little scared of her. The look in her eyes is like a crack addict. She's going to fight me any way she can to get these training pants. Instinct takes over and I run inside the bedroom where I lock the door behind me and slide down against it, crying but safe from the furious hammering.

I run to the bed, further from the pounding on the door. *Why is this happening?* This can't be what other parents go through? I lie on the bed, holding the training pants close to me, knowing she will not allow herself to have an accident.

I pray to God for help and guidance, holding the pull-up to the ceiling. Her rage turns into heavy crying, as the answer comes to me. I bring the diaper back down and breathe, using the tools Michi has given me. *I'm calm in the middle of the storm.*

*　　　*　　　*

I open the door and stand tall over my four-year-old Baby Jane, my arm stretched out, with the training pants held as high as it will go. "Do it in the potty and I will give you this pull-up."

She looks at it, a golden carrot above her head, then says, "I'll do it." She cries softly, as she goes into the bathroom and sits on the potty, fighting herself even as a strong pee stream pounds the water. The irony of using a pull-up to potty train Jani still hits me sometimes, years later.

I wait until she finishes then I let out a huge breath that I didn't even know I was holding inside me and fall to the floor, my arm shaking as I hand her the training pants. She's shaking too as she takes it from me and puts it on immediately.

"Wait until Daddy gets home!" I say, beaming with pride. I did it. SHE did it! We both did it and we both know it. Jani smiles at me and it's the first thing she tells Daddy when he gets home and he's equally shocked and excited.

Years later, I find out that Jani's 'irrational fear' was the shark she always saw swimming around inside toilets. An imaginary shark prevented her from sitting on the potty.

CHAPTER 4

THE BIRDCAGE

August 8th, 2007

It's Jani's 5th birthday, and I'm five months pregnant with Bodhi. Since this will be our last family trip for a while, we are spending it with Michael's dad and stepmom in Scottsdale, Arizona. Keeping Jani entertained is so hard, but at least she'll have a constant playmate soon. I can only pray that he gets her imagination.

Michael's stepmom is out getting her hair and nails done and I'm giving Michael time to play golf with his dad while I read to Jani on the front porch. Their gorgeous ranch-style home stretches half an acre with five rooms, including a playroom for the grandkids when they visit. There's even a guesthouse, but Jani still gets bored so easily.

"What are we going to do now, Mommy?" We've already been through the new books I just bought at the Barnes and Noble nearby. The bookstore patio has pop-up sprinklers in the ground that kept Jani entertained for a while.

"Do you want to go swimming?" I ask her.

"We already went swimming."

"I know, but we could do it again? Daddy should be home soon. Let's just wait for him. There are so many toys here that you haven't played with."

"Okay," Jani agrees and hops on a trike scooter, riding through the living room and into the kitchen. "I'm going to Kilimanjaro!"

"That's great, sweetie," I say and plop down on the couch, flipping channels as Michael's stepmom comes in. "Hi."

"Well, hi there," she responds in a civil-sweetness.

"Kilimanjaro, here I come!" Jani screeches along on the trike scooter she's outgrown but still enjoys riding on.

Michael's stepmom has tried talking with Jani before but it's never worked out too well. This time, she doesn't even try. She just turns around. "I'm going to lie down for a while. I've got a headache." Her sandals tap the floor, leading her to their bedroom. I hear the door to her room open, then close.

After too short a time, Jani is bored with the trike. Oh God, I have no idea how to pass the time and no one here to help. "Mommy," Jani gets off the scooter and stands up to me. "I feel like I'm living on the border between my world and the real world." Michael's stepmom is coming back into the living room, but I don't feel comfortable talking about this in front of her so I take Jani into the hallway.

"That's because you're so much smarter than most people." That's what we've always told her, and ourselves, even when our friends started suggesting we get her tested. Lynn's comment at the pool about Asperger's wasn't the first or the last. But she was so brilliant, just like Michael, and brilliant people don't usually fit in well. It was easier to keep believing that was all it was.

"I don't want to be smart!" Jani yells back at me.

"What do you mean? Being smart is a great thing. You are so lucky!"

"I don't feel lucky," she frowns. "I feel like I'm a bird trapped in a cage at Petco. I'm trying to find the combination to the lock so I can get out."

My mouth falls open. I'm at a loss for words. Usually, I can comfort Jani pretty easily, but I have no idea what to say about this. "It will get better," I promise her. "You're five years old today! You're going to have a brother. It will all get better."

"I want friends."

"I know you want friends."

"But they don't get my imagination."

"That's because you're more advanced than they are. As you get older, they'll catch up to you."

*   *   *

"Jani," Grandpa Bear and Michael come in, sweating from their golf game, "Nana and I want to take you shopping for your birthday."

"I need a shower first," Michael says, wiping the sweat from his brow.

"Well, so do I," his dad chuckles. "I'm saying after we shower, we'll go shopping, then out to dinner."

"I don't wanna go," Jani states, angrily.

"Are you being silly?" Grandpa says, in his kid-friendly voice. "You're five today. You can pick out whatever you want. We'll go to dinner and then come home and have cake!"

"NO! I don't want to go shopping!"

"Jani, we go to the mall all the time. You can pick out whatever you want," I plead with her.

"I'm NOT GOING!"

"Okay, if that's the way you want to be about it," Grandpa's adult voice returns "then we won't go." He marches off angrily.

"Dad, where are you going?"

"I'm going to take my shower, Mike. Then we're going to dinner. If she doesn't want to go shopping, I'm not going to force her to go shopping."

"Jani," Michael begs. "Why don't you want to go shopping? It's your birthday?"

"Don't give in like that, Mike. She's being a brat!" Michael and I look at each other, grateful we're not staying here long.

*   *   *

"Mike, she really needs to be in school," his dad says as we wait to be seated at the Olive Garden.

"We're still thinking about homeschooling Jani." I smile.

"She's doing okay," Michael insists while Jani dances around the waiting area. "She's way too advanced for kindergarten."

"Also, homeschooling will let us teach her at her own pace," I add.

"What a good boy he is," Michael's stepmom comments on a little boy waiting patiently. "He's cute too."

"I'm not talking about academics," his dad's frustration grows. "I'm talking about socialization!" Michael hates that word. It literally makes him cringe, like everything he's done to teach Jani is going to waste.

"Homeschooling isn't what it used to be. And if it doesn't work out we can still put her in regular kindergarten at Oak Hills. Kindergarten isn't mandatory," Michael tells his father, while Jani keeps wandering through the crowded house of people, finding her way up to the hostess and begging her for a table. "Look, I've got to start teaching her again."

Our buzzer sounds and the small red lights flash around it.

CHAPTER 5

CALL OF THE WILD

September 2007

We're on our way to the dog park when we pass an elementary school. I look at Jani through the rearview mirror. She sees the kids playing at recess. *She wants to be with them. I can tell by the look in her eyes.*

When we get to the dog park, we find the usual crowd of dog-sitters gathered in their white plastic chairs around a huge bucket of ice for the dogs to chew on. Jani plucks out the ice and spreads it around on the grass. "Please don't do that," one woman says. "The dogs like it in the bucket." Jani hand-claps. She's been told this so many times before but for whatever reason, it never sinks in. "Aren't you supposed to be in school?"

"I'm being homeschooled," Jani replies.

"Oh," is the woman's only response as she turns to pet her dog, then I turn to Jani.

"Jani, do you want to go to school? I mean, regular kindergarten? You are potty-trained now and it's only three and a half hours a day. You'd have other kids to play with...."

She looks up at me and then, "I don't want to go, but I think I need to. I need to be around them."

My jaw drops. "Okay. Then we'll do it! Right now! Honey!" I call our dog to come back thinking to myself. *For the first time in years, I'm going to get three and a half hours by myself, every weekday!*

We go straight to the administration office at our base school, Oak Hills, but Jani escapes my grip and flies into one of the offices while I'm talking with the secretary. "She can't go in there," the secretary tells me.

"I know," I sigh, then search out my daughter. "Jani! You have to come back here. It will only take a few minutes." I fetch her back and hold her close to me. "Is there anything else I need to do?"

"No, you filled out all the paperwork so you're all ready to go."

"We were going to homeschool, but I think it's good for her socialization that she tries out kindergarten." The secretary reassures me that I'm making a good decision and I breathe a sigh of relief. Three and a half hours of solitude. My time. My own time.

The only requirement is for Jani to get her TB shot. After that, it's her first day of kindergarten. I sit in the back, hoping I'll be able to leave soon, but I need to make sure everything goes okay first.

"January Schofield," the teacher calls out. All the kids are sitting in blue, green, yellow and red squares. Ugh. I told the teacher before class to call her Jani.

"NOT JANUARY!" she screams.

"You're not January?" the teacher asks. This is not going well.

"No, I'm…"

She's struggling and it hasn't even been five minutes. "She likes to be called Jani," I interrupt from the back of the room.

"Okay," the teacher agrees. "Jani." I sigh, relieved that's settled. I'd made a deal with Jani: She had to pick a name and stick with it.

"Today we're going to read a story…" her teacher starts out.

Oh God, there's no way Jani's going to make it through this. I see her looking around at the other kids. They're entranced with the story already and Jani simply isn't. Damn it.

* * *

"January Schofield!" The teacher assistant calls her over to another desk for testing.

"NOT JANUARY!" Jani shrill-screams once again at the top of her lungs. Apparently, the assistant didn't hear us the first time because she was working with the other kids.

"I need her over here for academic testing," she looks directly at me now.

"Jani, you need to go over there."

Jani goes over and completes the testing on her colors, letters, numbers, and shapes. "Now, I need you to write out your full name here."

"I'm not writing January!"

"You have too. It's on your school records," the assistant insists, tone now matching Jani's adult-speak.

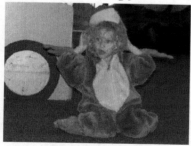

"But I'm not January. I'm Hot Dog." This is Jani's newest name, but it isn't like Blue-Eyed Tree Frog or even Wednesday. When she calls herself Blue-Eyed Tree Frog, she's having fun and playing. When she says she's Wednesday, she's getting mad but she's still mostly in our world. "Hot Dog" is different, and not in a good way. The teacher's assistant signals for me to come over.

Jani, the blue-eyed tree frog.

"She's going to need to write her name in the space here by the end of the school year or she won't pass kindergarten," the assistant looks straight into her eyes.

"What? You're kidding me!"

"She needs to be able to write her name. Also, a lot of these kids here don't speak English as a first language," she tells Jani. "They're going to get confused."

"Can't she just write Jani?" I am begging.

"Her records show January."

"I'm NOT JANUARY!" Jani throws down the chair and storms toward the door.

"She's way too 'out-of-the-box' for this class," I weeble-wobble after her. "I'm just sorry I brought her here in the first place. It was my mistake."

The assistant follows me out. "You didn't make a mistake," she walks quickly alongside me. "She needs to be here."

"She's a genius. She did the work these kids are doing when she was two years old!"

"If you're sure you want to do this?"

"Do I have a choice? My daughter loves to learn but she's not going to learn anything in this classroom."

"How to interact with other kids her own age."

"I'm just going to homeschool her," I say, disappointed that I'll be losing those three and a half hours. I go back to the school secretary and hand her the packet. "It's not working out."

She sighs. "I'll keep her file here in case you change your mind."

"Okay, but I'm going to homeschool her," I say, determined. When we get to the car, I'm at loss. I have no idea where to go from here.

"Can we see Grace today?"

Hmmm. "Maybe," I think for a moment. Jani's right. I should call Michi, Grace's mom. I just hope she's home. "Hold on, I'm calling her right now," I tell Jani. Thank God, she answers. "We've decided on homeschooling."

"Bad experience with school?"

"They're just not ready for 'out-of-the-box' thinkers. Can we come over?" I am desperate.

"Sure."

"Thank you."

Jani and Grace play while Michi works with me on my breathing. "You're overwhelmed."

"I know I'm overwhelmed! Michael's teaching all the time, and Jani's just being 'Jani' and I really don't know where to put her. I'm in my third trimester and all the kids she's played with for years are in school so I don't even see my moms' group anymore."

Michi listens with intent, hearing every word I say before she responds. After all, she is a professional Life Coach. Since we're friends, she helps me for free. "First we have to work on you. You have to use your breathing tools more effectively. If *you're* calm, then *she'll* be calm. And remember, *love wins*. No matter what she's going through, you have to be strong."

"I don't feel strong enough." Hormonal tears break through.

"You will. Feel the muscles in my stomach." Michi has a fifty-year-old body that a twenty-year-old would envy. She is pure strength. She loosens her muscles and stands in front of me. "Try to push me down. Go ahead, just try to push me down." She is daring me.

"Okay," I say, and try to push her down and she stumbles a bit.

"Did you see that? I was off-balance. I was not like a tree firmly rooted in the ground." She straightens her posture, inhales, then exhales. "Now try to push me down."

I do the same thing, but Michi doesn't move this time.

"Try harder."

I try harder to push her down. She still doesn't budge an inch. "That's incredible."

"That's what I'm talking about. You always need to carry your posture tall and strong like a firmly rooted tree, especially when you're in the 'eye' of the storm. Remember, 'Keep Calm in the Middle of the Storm.'" Michi had invited me to hear her speak at the Bodhi Tree Bookstore, which is when I chose the name Bodhi for our son. It means enlightened, awakened.

"I can do that," I stand tall and proud.

"I know you can do that," she says, then turns serious. "Grace, what are you two doing? Remember, you're going to need to do your homework on the computer."

Jani and Grace fly downstairs for a moment, "Ta-da!" Grace shows off her Jani-doll in full-on make-up. Even her hair is done up beautifully, with little curls around her face. "We're playing dress-up!" Grace says, and bringing Jani back upstairs.

"She looks beautiful Grace and so do you! Thank you." I still have tears in my eyes. I look at Michi. "I'm really hormonal."

"I know you are," she hugs me.

*   *   *

By October, I am out of places to take Jani. I even try a home-schooling network that's really big in Valencia, but it doesn't work either. Jani won't sit in a formal or informal class of any kind. So, we're back at the dog park.

"Time for Dog Class!" Jani shouts to the dogs, branches of tree sticks held high above her head. The dogs come running up and Jani throws the sticks into the air. Honey and the other dogs who decided to attend the class chase their stick of choice, then plop down on the grass and gnaw on it.

A Husky puppy comes late to the game, and bounds up to her, knocking her down. Jani's been inside the dog park her entire life so she usually just gets up quickly, brushes herself off and continues playing, but this time her face darkens.

"Are you alright?" A man in his early thirties approaches, offering her a hand up.

"She's fine," I tell him from the bench where I've plopped down. "Our dog Honey always jumps on her," I point to where Honey's exploring.

"BAD DOG!" Jani yells at the husky puppy. Huh? "You're a BAD DOG!" She picks up a fallen tree branch and waves it above her head like she's going to hit this dog.

"Jani, what are you doing? That's a husky puppy." She doesn't answer me. She just stares at the dog.

"I'm sorry. She didn't mean to jump on her."

"No, it's okay. Jani's not usually like this." Watching her, this grown man is clearly afraid, steering his dog away from her.

"Jani, come here." No answer. Instead, she runs after the man and his dog, still carrying the stick above her head, repeating the phrase "bad dog." The man and his dog are now running away from my five-year-old daughter, while I waddle as fast as I can after her. When I catch up to her I grab the stick out of her hand and apologize to the man. "My daughter is not usually like this. I'm having a baby so I think she's just adjusting to it."

His eyes are fearful though. This is a grown man. How can he be afraid of my five-year-old daughter? What does he see when he looks at her? I turn my attention back to Jani. "We're going right now!" I tell her.

"She's a bad dog," Jani keeps repeating.

"Jani, you can't hit dogs! I won't be able to bring you here anymore."

"I don't want to come to the dog park anymore!"

CHAPTER 6

SWEET REINDEER

November 2007

"What's 300 plus 100?" Jani asks on our elevator ride up to Dr. Matz's office. It's the same office I visited when I was pregnant with Jani.

"400," I answer, just as the elevator door opens and I see the number 400 staring back at me.

"I told you it was 400," Jani jokes. She comes with me as I go into the bathroom for my urine test. "Where does it go?" she asks as I slide my specimen through the small window.

"To the lab."

"What do they do with it in the lab?"

"They test for things like diabetes and iron levels." I've never really thought about it, but I think I read that somewhere. We're waiting in the waiting room as the receptionist walks back to her desk. She remembers all the way back to when I was pregnant with Jani. In fact, most of the same staff from five years ago is still here.

"Hi, January," she says, as sweet as Apple Pie.

Oh no.

"NOT JANUARY!"

"Jani, stop it!" I'm losing my patience. I hate to keep explaining this to everyone. Maybe my mom was right about letting her get away with everything after all. "She likes to be called Jani," I tell her.

The same nurse who made sure I had enough prenatal vitamins for Jani so long ago hears Jani's vicious scream and says, "So, you've managed to spoil your daughter."

"Yeah, she's spoiled," I agree. What else can I say? Jani *is* acting like a spoiled brat.

"Alright," she nods her head back and forth then leads us into the examining room. "Dr. Matz will be right with you."

I get up on the table while Jani walks in circles around the room. She has her Leap Frog to entertain her, but she's just not interested anymore. She starts investigating the equipment, including the ultrasound machine. She pushes some buttons and starts jerking things around.

"Don't touch," I whisper-warn her. She stops playing with the machine but walks out the door. "Jani, you can't leave! You need to come back here!" I manage to heave myself off the examining table to pursue my daughter as she heads into Dr. Matz's office and starts rearranging the furniture. I know Dr. Matz is going to be upset, but I'm about to pop and I can't physically do anything to remove her.

Be calm in the middle of the storm, I tell myself, walking back over to Apple Pie at her receptionist desk. "Uh, could you help you with something?"

"Okay," she looks at me, a bit baffled, as I bring her over to Dr. Matz's office. At this point, Jani is crawling under Dr. Matz's desk and going through her files. Apple's jaw drops. "She can't be doing this!"

"I know, but I can't physically remove her and she's not listening to me."

Apple Pie looks at my big belly and sighs. "Jani, Dr. Matz is going to be really angry. She doesn't like anyone getting into her stuff."

No answer.

I crawl down on my knees and grab her by the back of her shirt. "You need to come with me!"

"NO!"

"Why aren't you listening to your mother?" Apple asks.

I lose my grip on her and she pulls a box of papers down, splattering them all around the office. DAMN IT! Apple leaves just as I start cleaning up the mess Jani's still making. Dr. Matz stares down at me from the door to her office. "I can see you now." Her voice is as cold as ice.

She goes through the motions of my exam as quickly as humanly possible while I hold Jani firmly at my side as she twists around, pushing buttons on the ultrasound machine. "What did you just do?!" Dr. Matz fiddles around with the machine. "I think you just broke it! Don't touch it again!" Jani doesn't respond.

Dr. Matz turns to me. "I'll see you next month for delivery."

"That's it?" I ask her. Usually, Dr. Matz invites me back into her office to discuss what happens next.

"That's it," she says abruptly, walking me out of the examining room, Jani by my side. "And don't ever bring your daughter back into my office again."

I swallow hard. This is the doctor who brought Jani into this world. Shouldn't she have a special feeling since she delivered Jani into my arms five years ago? I don't get how she can be like this. I call Michael on the way home. "Jani got kicked out of Dr. Matz's office," I say loud enough for Jani to hear and make Michael upset.

"What?! Can you hold on for a minute?" I hate bothering Michael at work, but I don't know who else to call about this. "Okay," he's calm. "I just needed to get out of the office to hear what you're saying."

"I'm saying that Jani pretty much broke Dr. Matz's ultrasound machine, then she messed up her office, throwing all her files around, and now they don't want her back there ever again. So, from now on *you're* going to have to take her whenever I have appointments. I'm not going through this again!"

"Why are you yelling at me?!"

"I'm angry!"

"I know you're angry, but I'm working!"

"I know you're working and I'm sorry for calling you, but I can't do this anymore!"

"Look," Michael's voice returns to the calm, cool, collected manner he maintains at work, "You're almost done being pregnant and we're *not* doing this again!"

"I know!" I wipe tears from my eyes.

"I'm almost done teaching for the semester. If you have to go to the doctor again, I'll just take Jani to school with me."

I turn back to Jani. "Whenever I have a doctor's appointment Daddy is going to take you to work with him since you can't be civilized in a doctor's office or anywhere else!"

"You're being mean to her," Michael scolds me over the phone.

"I know that! I'm just so tired of this."

"I've gotta get back to work."

"Fine." I hang up and cry.

"I can't help it," Jani speaks up from her car seat and I turn around to face her. "My mind is going like this," she rolls one of her wrists over the other at warped speed. She's always had the autistic trait of hand-flapping, but this is different. "Most peoples' are going like this," she continues, slow-motioning her wrist-roll rock-slamming.

I feel guilty already. "I'm sorry. I know your mind is going so fast. That's just because you're extremely smart and people don't appreciate it. I'm sorry," I apologize again.

* * *

"Thanks for meeting us," I tell Bethanne when we get to Travel Town, a train museum near the LA Zoo.

"Brandon never turns down a playdate at Travel Town." We let the kids explore the stationary trains. One minute, they're sitting on the train across from each other. The next minute they're hanging off the engine, laughing and having fun.

"We only have a few friends left now and it's getting harder for me to move around."

"Well, you know what I think," Bethanne starts out.

"We've already tried regular school and it didn't work out. Then I went to homeschooling and that didn't work either. It's the kids. They don't 'get' her imagination."

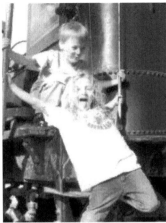

"At 146, Jani is profoundly gifted. That is as far from 'normal' as a kid who is severely mentally challenged. They should call it 'severely gifted'."

Jani and Brandon hanging out at Travel Town.

"That is so true. There are so few friends I can find for her."

We look over at Jani and Brandon. They're walking toward a gated-off nativity scene. It's set up to be seen from the little train that runs around the outside of the museum so the back of the scene is toward us. Jani tugs at the gate, trying to get inside.

"She's testing you, isn't she?"

"Yeah," I admit. "And I don't have the energy."

"Jani, the sign says you can't go in there," Bethanne cautions, while Brandon is deciding if he should follow Jani's lead or listen to his mother. "And Brandon, don't even think about it."

Jani slips through the gate. It isn't exactly locked up tight and my little girl slips through easily.

"Jani!" Bethanne roars. "You CANNOT go through there!" She turns to me. "Do you want me to get her?"

"Please," I say, exhausted from the weight I'm carrying inside my stomach and on my shoulders. Brandon runs over to me and I pat him on the head. He's so easy to take care of.

Bethanne trespasses through the gate then calls over to me. "You know, if they really want to keep people out, they need to do a way better job." I continue to pat Brandon on the head as Bethanne makes her way over to Jani petting Rudolph the Reindeer. "Jani, you're breaking and entering," she says, sternly.

"I'm petting Rudolph," Jani tilts her head to the side. "He's so sweet."

"Should I call the Security Guard, or are you going to come out?" No response, just more petting Rudolph. "Fine," Bethanne retreats back out through the gate, clearly on a mission now. "Can you watch Brandon for me?"

"Sure." Could there be anything easier?

"Why is Jani acting like this?" Brandon asks me.

"I don't know, Brandon," I answer, wistfully trying to forget why I'm even having this conversation with a five-year-old. "I guess she's just dealing with a life changing event, becoming a big sister. You know." Brandon's little brother is almost two so I figure he could relate to this, but he doesn't say anything. He just sits by me as we both watch Jani hover over Rudolph the Reindeer.

Bethanne marches back just ahead of the security guard. He looks more like a guy hanging around the place than an actual authority figure. Nonetheless, he's got the key to the gate. Walking through an open gate is easier than squeezing through the opening, especially while carrying a four-year-old.

He opens it and looks over at Bethanne. "So, what do you want me to do?"

"I want you to escort her out of here," Bethanne is fuming as she leads him over to Jani.

"Sweet reindeer," Jani is now swaying back and forth, petting Rudolph's back.

"You want me to physically pick her up and move her?" he squint-eyes Bethanne.

"YES!"

"Ohhhh," he puts his hands up like he's about to be arrested. "I can't do that!"

"Susan," Bethanne sighs in pure anger and frustration. "Do you want me to just pick her up and go?"

"Sure," I sigh. "I'll take Brandon."

Bethanne bats the guard away. "Never mind." He shrugs and leaves the trespassers inside the gate. Once Bethanne picks her up, Jani doesn't fight being carried to the car, even though she usually hates being carried.

"Sometimes I think you would be a better mom to Jani than I am," I tell her after she's put Jani back in her car seat while Brandon peacefully waits at my side.

"I'm not with her 24 hours a day," Bethanne says, her own patience wearing thin. "Jani's just...Jani. She's got a mind of her own, and it's certainly out of this world. But I do find her interesting, even admirable at times."

"So do I. She's just really hard to raise."

"I'd agree with that."

CHAPTER 7

I SURRENDER

December 17th, 2007, 8:30 am

Dr. Matz comes in to check on me and says the magic words. "If I pop the bag now it will be within an hour or two."

"Let's do it," I tell her, then immediately call Michael.

"I'll be right there." His voice is stressed. He and Jani are staying at a nearby hotel with his parents. As I'd expected, things did not go too well with them last night. They never do when Jani is involved, but what could I do? I'm kind of tied up right now.

"How's Jani?" I ask, a bit concerned but still excited over my new son's impending arrival.

"Okay," he says, but his voice is telling another story: Not bad, but not good.

"Don't forget to bring the camera! I want Bodhi's birth on film just like we did with Jani."

"I know. I've got it."

*　　　*　　　*

At 9:33 am, our Bodhi Schofield arrives much the same way Jani did, without Dr. Matz needing to use a vacuum at the last minute this time. "This will be your easy one," she predicts as Bodhi comes out, with a loud wail. He stops short at this as though he just heard he's supposed to be the 'easy one.'

Michael cuts the umbilical cord, handing it over to Dr. Matz who quickly puts it into a stem cell kit to be stored in Florida. "At least we know he's okay," I say in response to his quick scream coming out.

"Sounds good." Dr. Matz smiles, forgiveness on her face.

*   *   *

Michael and I are snuggling with Bodhi when his dad calls. "What's going on?" I ask as a dark shadow comes over Michael's face. Our moments of shared bonding time with Bodhi are just that, moments.

"Nothing," Michael shakes head, clearly upset over something.

"What is it? Is Jani okay?"

"They're fighting with her."

"What?! I thought they were going to take her some place fun so we could have time...."

"They were!" Now he's the one yelling. "But you don't know what happened last night."

"What happened last night?" Before he tells me I rush to judgment. "I should have gone with my instincts and had her sleep over at Michi's so she could be with Grace."

"Yeah, well, it's too late now." Michael turns on me.

"What is it?!"

"She was acting up last night. It was horrible. They're going to bring her here and take the next flight home."

"But I'm still in the hospital!"

"Look, they can't handle it. She's being a brat and they're going home!"

"Fine. I'll call Michi."

*   *   *

Michael's parents bring Jani to the hospital. She's wearing the same clothes she was in the day before. Michael's dad checks Bodhi to make sure he's a Schofield, takes some photos, and they're off. Since his stepmom has "a bad migraine," she doesn't even enter the hospital.

*   *   *

It's pouring rain by the time Michael brings Michi up to my room. "They won't let Grace come up," he says. "She's still too young."

Michi immediately looks at Bodhi. "Oh, he's beautiful."

I try to forget all the chaos going on around me and focus in on the moment. "Can you take Jani overnight? Michael's supposed to help Dr. Matz with Bodhi's circumcision, but he can't do it if we don't have someone to watch Jani." I'm begging.

"Sure, we can take her," Michi smiles, snuggling Bodhi in her arms. "What happened to Michael's parents?"

"They couldn't handle Jani and his stepmom was having bad migraines."

"They're not equipped," she says.

Michael comes back in with Jani's suitcase. "I just checked the lobby. Grace and Jani are doing okay." He turns to Michi. "All Jani's clothes are packed in here."

"I knew I should have had her stay with you. I made a big mistake. Michael told me his stepmom slapped her for picking her nose and then Jani slapped her back and they got into a slap fight."

"They tried, okay?" Michael's defenses are up, but I hear disappointment cracking in his voice.

"I really appreciate you coming out here, Michi. Jani will too."

Dr. Matz comes into my room, handing Michael his scrubs. "We're getting ready to do the circumcision."

"We should be going then," Michi hands Bodhi back to me, "before the rain gets too bad."

"Thank you." I am crying, again.

"It's our pleasure." Michi gives me a warm hug then takes Jani's bag downstairs, where the girls are waiting.

A few minutes later, Michael comes into my room, dressed in scrubs, ready to help Dr. Matz with Bodhi's circumcision. I smile at Michael. For the first time, I'm able to relax in my hospital bed, relieved because he's with Bodhi and Jani's with Michi and Grace. I am thinking about Bodhi going through his circumcision when the phone rings. It's Michi. I know they're driving in the rain and it's only been a half hour since they left the hospital.

"Is everything okay?"

"Yeah, we're okay," she pauses. "Now."

"Now? What do you mean? Did you get into an accident?! Is Jani okay?"

"No, no. It's not that. Jani's fine. It's just that," she stammers, "we had an incident."

"An incident?"

"Jani bit Grace."

"What?!"

"She was having a meltdown and I was driving. She was kicking my seat and I told her to stop and she...she attacked Grace."

"She attacked, Grace?!" My breath stops. "Is Grace okay?"

"Yes, she was just startled. It came out of nowhere. But I'm so proud of Grace for using her FunZen tools. She didn't react. She worked to calm Jani down instead."

"I'm so sorry," I apologize. "Jani has *never* done that before!"

"It's okay, but could you have Michael come over to our house and take her home with him? I don't think it's the best time for a sleepover."

"I understand," I say, gulping hard air. "Michael is still in with Dr. Matz but as soon as he's done I'll send him over."

Michael comes out of the circumcision, his palms all sweaty. "That was intense."

"Is Bodhi okay?" I'm so used to asking about Jani that it's weird to hear myself asking about Bodhi now.

"Yeah," Michael perks up. "He just had a surprised look on his face, but he didn't really cry or anything. I held his hand all the way through it."

"I'm so glad you were there." Tears flood my eyes.

"Good job," Dr. Matz walks in and pats him on his shoulder.

"Thanks. You did a great job, too," he returns the compliment. She smiles at him before turning to me. "How are you feeling?"

"Okay."

"Any pain or anything like that?"

"No," I tell her, although in a strange way I don't feel connected to my body right now.

"Good," she smiles, then takes off her gloves and heads out of the room.

"Michi called..." I start off to Michael. "Jani bit Grace on their way home."

"She bit Grace?!"

"Yeah. I don't know why and neither do Michi or Grace. Michi said Jani had a meltdown and bit Grace. She wants you to take her home. She doesn't think it's the right time for a sleepover."

Michael's face drops. "It was going to be our night with Bodhi."

"I know. I guess it's just not meant to be."

"I'm not getting to spend any time with my son," Michael rightly complains.

"It's just hard right now. She's the older sibling, just like my brother was. You're an only child so you never had to go through this. Remember, my mom said my brother twisted his hair out when I was born. It will get easier. We'll all be at home soon."

The next morning, Bodhi is sitting by my side, watching television. It's like he's already grown up in a weird sort of way. I get up with him and show him the trees like I remember my mom's mother, Grandma Rae, doing with me when I was little. Sure enough, he sees them. He's alert, just like Jani was after she was born. He's ready to learn, but in a little calmer, more relaxed way. He's actually happy and content to just be in my arms.

The phone rings and I bring Bodhi back to bed with me. "Is Jani up for a visit?" It's Bethanne.

"*Yes.* Please!! But wait..." I remember what Michael said yesterday. "Brandon can't come upstairs to my room."

"That's okay. We want to take Jani for a playdate at Orcutt Ranch. We can be there around one o'clock."

"Perfect. Michael will be back with Jani."

"Aren't your in-laws taking care of her?"

"No, they left early. They couldn't handle her." Our moms' group used to take the kids on nature walks at Orcutt. It's near the hospital and Jani's always liked it. "I think that would be perfect. She's having a hard time right now. She bit Grace last night."

"Oh, wow. You know, Brandon struggled a bit when his brother was born. It's hard for them, but I think Jani will be okay with us. We'll pick some lemons."

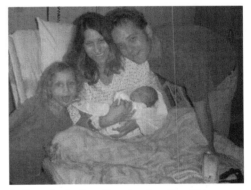

I'm relieved that Bethanne isn't scared off. Michael and I finally have a few hours alone with Bodhi, taking turns feeding and diapering our new son. My breasts have always been very sensitive and I fear breastfeeding. With Jani, my milk never came in. I know that now because my good friend Marilyn, who has four kids, told me that I would know when I was engorged, but I could never figure out what she meant. Until now. My breasts are huge and leaking. I feel guilty, but, I'm still scared to breastfeed, so Michael and I take turns giving Bodhi his bottle.

The whole family the day Bodhi was born.

Bodhi pees in Michael's face as he changes his diaper. Michael laughs and wipes his mouth. "I forgot about this. Something new to get used to."

"Yeah, it happened to me too. I was thinking the same thing."

"He's such a cute little guy," Michael finishes diapering him and starts nuzzling him close.

"Yes, he is."

When Jani comes back with Bethanne, I'm scared to ask how everything went, but they're all wearing smiles and holding lemons. "Everything went fine," Bethanne is happy to report. "They both picked lemons and I even gave Jani a quick hug and told her, 'I love you, Jani.' I know how much she hates being held, so I made it quick and she was okay with it."

"Thank you, Bethanne," I burst into tears again. Bethanne talks so much like a computer sometimes, but that really resonates with Jani and she's one of the very few people who can do that.

"Brandon had a hard time when his brother was born too. He had so many health problems that I had to spend a lot of time in the hospital with him. Brandon got the short end of the stick. But now he loves him."

I smile. There is hope for our future. We just have to hang on.

*　　　*　　　*

Two days later, I'm in the middle of being discharged when Michael blasts in. "I can't find Jani!"

"Please lower your voice. Bodhi's right over there," I whisper, nodding over to my little guy, asleep in his infant car carrier.

"I know," Michael says through gritted teeth, "but we can't leave the hospital without Jani." Before Bodhi was born I'd gone on my own to Toys "R" Us and found this beautiful light green infant outfit I wanted to put him in. I love him so much. *God, why is this happening?*"

"I'm aware of that. I just want you to be a bit calmer." I pick Bodhi up and bring him back to bed with me.

"I can't be calmer!" He yells at me. "You have no idea what it's been like this week with you in the hospital."

"What?!"

"She's been running around the nurse's station and I lost her again!"

A nurse comes into my room along with a new pediatrician. "Your daughter can't be running around the nurses' station," she scolds us, as if we don't already know that.

"I know. I know, alright," Michael snaps back, running out of the room to find Jani.

"Bodhi checked out perfectly," the pediatrician looks down at us. "I feel sorry for you." I clutch my son to me as tears stream down my cheeks, but no words come.

The doctor turns to leave and I nestle Bodhi closer, surrendering myself to God. Bodhi wasn't supposed to come into the world like this. I was a second sibling just like him and it's not fair. We should be happy and joyful, enjoying our new baby. Instead, we're in hell.

I let out a mournful breath, trying desperately to comprehend how we got here. I gave birth two days ago, to a baby we both desperately wanted and my husband is yelling at me because our five-year-old daughter is out of control. I decide not to say a word. Even though I was the one who gave birth, he had the harder job because he was responsible for taking care of Jani, alone. Usually, we give each other breaks, but it's been a non-stop nightmare for him since Sunday night.

"Now STAY HERE!" Michael angrily jerks Jani back into my hospital room, slamming the door behind him, as I put Bodhi back in his infant carrier.

"I want to go! NOW!" Jani screams back at him.

"We can't go yet!" I tell her, grabbing my camera off the nightstand. I need to take a picture of Bodhi in his going home outfit. I really wish I could enjoy this moment but it's not possible. I'll appreciate the picture in the future.

The nurse comes back in. "You need to follow procedure before we discharge you."

"I know."

"We're bringing in the wheelchair now. Put the car seat on your lap and your husband and daughter will walk alongside you." I actually remember the procedure from when Jani was born but it was so much easier with just one.

As she leaves the room, I turn to Jani. "Jani, you need to just stay here. We're going to go home now. They're just getting me a wheelchair."

"Do we have everything?" Michael combs through the closets and bathroom, then under the bed.

"I think so. I started packing last night."

Jani tries to run again, but this time I grab her, holding her tightly on my lap. She tilts her head, looking above the door on my left side and in a witchy high-pitched voice, I've never heard before, squeals, "Oooh, she's not pregnant anymoorre." I turn to the door and stare at it. It's closed. There's no one there. I let Jani slip off my lap and sit in shock.

The door opens. "Are we all ready now?" The nurse asks, bringing in a wheelchair.

"Yes, we're trying here," I bravely tell her. "We just need help…" I start to choke up "with our daughter."

"Hyperactive, huh?"

"Yeah. We had her tested for Asperger's, but she doesn't have that."

"It's probably ADHD," she says, more empathetic this time. "You should see a doctor and have her checked out."

"We will." With everything that's been happening, I am about to keel over.

CHAPTER 8

CAN'T YOU DO SOMETHING?

December 2007

"Can't you DO something?!" Michael screams at me from the bathroom. He's struggling to keep Jani's legs in one place. She's kicking at him like a bike rider in a marathon. Earlier, she was in the closet asking how she could break her own neck.

"I can't control this!" Jani cries.

"What do you want me to do?!" My voice is a harsh whisper. "Bodhi's asleep." He's only a few days old.

"Call Michi. Maybe she and Grace can come over and help."

"Okay," I shut the bathroom door.

"Michi!" I'm relieved to get her on the phone right away. "I need your help. Jani's going crazy over here!"

"You should take her to the hospital," Michi says.

Huh? "She's not hurt. Why would I take her to the hospital?"

"There are places for kids like that."

"What are you talking about?"

"For kids who are out of control, like Jani."

"But she's just five."

"They have five-year-olds there."

"You're serious?! How do you know this?"

"I spent time inside a mental health facility. I know about these places."

My mind flashes back to my dad's mom, Grandma Freda getting electric shock treatments for depression. She had periodic "nervous breakdowns" throughout his life. She had a four-year-old son who somehow burned to death in the kitchen. She was never the same after that. No one knows exactly how it happened, but my dad became what he refers to as the 'replacement' child. Grandma Freda's brother Henry had schizophrenia and lived at Napa State Hospital for most of his life. Every time he was released he would just run and they'd have to bring him back.

My legs are collapsing under my knees, so I use my free hand to steady my arm on the kitchen counter. "Michi, can you hold on?"

"Sure."

My head is dizzy and my breathing is shallow as I call out to Michael. "Michi says we need to take her to the hospital." I start to cry. She's still my baby girl.

Michael opens the bathroom door as Jani starts to settle down. "She's right." Why do I feel like both Michi and Michael are in a class way above my head? "What hospital will take her?"

"What hospital…" I turn back to the phone, repeating Michael's question to Michi.

"Henry Mayo. They should have a children's ward there." The oxygen is leaving my brain. I'm about to faint. "Susan, are you there?"

"I can't do this. Oh, my God. What is happening, Michi?" I'm crying harder.

"Just do what I say and get her to the hospital. They have to take her to the Emergency Room. They're open 24 hours."

"It's okay now!" Michael calls out. "Jani's calmed down. We got through it."

"Oh thank God. They got through it," I tell Michi over the

60

phone as Michael comes out into the kitchen.

"That's good. Just call me later, Susan."

"I will," I promise Michi, hang up, then turn to Michael. "So, we need to take her to a doctor."

"Not a physical doctor. She needs a psychiatrist," he clarifies. I crumble to the floor, crying uncontrollably.

*   *   *

We make it through Christmas, barely. After calling everyone in Michael's insurance network, we're lucky and find one child psychologist on such short notice. She happens to be Michael's own psychologist's partner. As soon as we tell her we have a new baby, she sees us the next day, then immediately refers us to Dr. Howe, a child psychiatrist, who makes an emergency appointment. This is the first time, but not the last, that having an infant in our home makes "them" pay attention to Jani.

"You both need to sign this for me to prescribe treatment," Dr. Howe hands Michael some papers. Michael signs his name and hands it over to me.

"What's this?"

"You have to sign it for Jani to get medication," he says.

"What does she have?"

Dr. Howe looks at me, quizzically, then says, "Anxiety."

"Ahhh," I sigh. "Of course, that makes so much sense since we just had a baby." I sign the paper.

Dr. Howe takes the form from us as Jani is content playing with the dollhouse in her office. "Now, I need to know about your family histories."

Michael talks about how he was on Ritalin for ADHD as a child, for uncontrollable rages. She nods, unsurprised. Then, I tell her about my family, going back in time a bit to explain about my dad's side of the family, my grandmother and her brother. Dr. Howe finishes the family history. "Okay, I'm going to get samples of Risperdal. That treats anxiety."

But as she goes to the door, I stop her. "I mean, it couldn't be anything else, could it? Like what my great-uncle had? Like schizophrenia?"

"No!" she whips the words back at me like I'm a child who just swore at her. "We're not going there. We are *not* going there."

"Okay. Okay!" I hold up my white flag, no harm done. After all, I was just asking.

Dr. Howe comes back with the samples of Risperdal and asks Jani to come sit next to her. Amazingly, Jani follows her orders. "Can you swallow a pill?"

"Yes," Jani answers, seriously, as she plays with the sleeve of her lavender sweater. It is out of shape and sopping wet from her constant chewing. She takes the pill from Dr. Howe and swallows it.

"You can go back to playing with the dollhouse now." And Jani does just that, numbering the dolls 72 and 73. "She's got a thing for numbers, huh?"

"Yeah," I say. "She can even count to a thousand. Here's her IQ test." I always carry it in my purse as a source of pride.

Dr. Howe glances at it and tosses it to the side. "I know she's intelligent. That's not the problem." While the doctor watches Jani to see if she has any reaction to the medication, we finish discussing our family histories. After about fifteen minutes, Dr. Howe swivels her chair back to Jani, still engaged with the dollhouse. "How do you feel, Jani?"

"Good," she answers. Her sweater is dry although the cuff is permanently crinkled, but she is definitely calmer. "Can we go to CPK?" I look over at Michael.

"Sure. We may as well try it out now." I nod to them both and tuck the sample pills away in my purse.

"You can give her another dose in an hour, if needed," Dr. Howe tells us. "My guess is that we'll probably have to raise it anyway."

*   *   *

It's the dinner rush at CPK. We usually avoid evenings because the last thing we need is to be chasing Jani through a crowd of people while she screams "I'm sixteen! I'm working!" We always end up next to the chefs preparing the pizza by the fire.

Michael entertains Jani with the kid's menu. I have no idea what I would do without him. I look over at Bodhi resting peacefully in his car seat. It is a moment to appreciate.

Then Jani gets up from her chair and looks around. *Uh-oh…* "Jani, do you need another Risperdal?"

"Yes," she tells me, straightforward. As I reach into my purse, she eyes the fire blazing in the oven and says, "You know, I would be running over there right now, but I'm controlling it."

My jaw drops as I give her the next dosage of Risperdal. Tears of relief run down my cheeks. We did the right thing.

CHAPTER 9

WELCOME TO HOLLAND

January 2008

In 1987 Emily Perl Kingsley wrote a poem. She was always being asked to describe what her experiences raising a child with a disability were like. She metaphorically illustrates this by comparing a pre-planned move to Italy. You've already learned some of the language and know the places you want to go when you get settled there. But then your plane is detoured in mid-flight—to Holland. And there you will stay. You wonder, what happened? This must be a mistake because this was not the place you intended to go and you mourn that loss, but if you continue to do that, you'll never fully enjoy all Holland has to offer.

I found this out for myself back in January 2008 when Jani was diagnosed with anxiety and Bodhi was nearly one month old.

*   *   *

God, please get me to the zoo! I'm going as fast as the freeway speed limit allows. The LA Zoo is in Griffith Park, just beyond Burbank. I thought I could do this. I even calculated the time. It would only be a 30-minute straight drive from Valencia to the zoo, but

Bodhi's crying again. We've already learned that he hates car rides, but what am I supposed to do? A lot of our friends and favorite play spaces are still in "The Valley" and it takes time to drive there from Valencia. Michael's at work today but at least we have a playdate.

"I can't stand his crying!" Jani plugs her ears, letting out an ear-piercing scream of her own.

"Just put the bottle in his mouth," I order her, driving south past the Burbank exit. *Thank God we're almost there. Only a few more exits.* She puts the bottle in his mouth but he spits it back out and continues to wail. "I think he's got gas," I tell her.

"AAAAAHHHHHHHHHHH!" she yells in his face and his eyes open wider than ever. He looks like he's in shock. *Dammit! Why did I ever think I could do this?*

My cell rings. It's Lynn, "Are you here? I can't find you."

"I'm not there yet," I tell Lynn, frantic.

"Is everything okay?" Now she sounds concerned.

"Bodhi won't stop crying and Jani's screaming," I tell her, then turn back to Jani. I allowed her in the back seat with Bodhi only because she's on her Risperdal now and she promised she'd help me get to the zoo. "What are you doing?!" I see Jani taking off her seat-belt. "NO!"

"What's happening?" Lynn asks, like hearing a police chase on the radio.

"Jani's taking her seatbelt off."

"My girls do that all the time," Lynn calmly reflects.

"No, this is different," I say, defeated.

Jani jumps over the seat and starts shifting gears around. I end the call and shove her back. "Are you CRAZY?! I could have an accident here. Get back there! And stay back there!" The phone rings. It's Lynn again. "I don't know if we're going to make it today," I cry, then turn back to Jani. "Do you *want* to go to the zoo?!"

She takes off her shoe and tosses it at me.

"It sounds like you're having a hard time getting here and the parking is horrible. Should we just meet at Shane's Inspiration instead?" Shane's Inspiration is a playground near the zoo.

Bodhi's cry gets weaker as he drifts off to sleep. "No, just stay there for now," I tell her, missing the turn-off. "FUCK! I missed the exit! Just please stay there!" Now Jani is throwing paper at me from the backseat.

Lynn sounds as rushed as I feel. "We'll just wait till you get here. I have a beautiful baby gift for Bodhi."

"Thank you." An empty box strikes the back of my head as I keep an eye on the road, my hand searching my purse for another Risperdal. I spin the car around, hitting traffic from the other direction. "Jani. You need to take this RIGHT NOW!" I push it into her mouth. "Here's your water," I toss a bottle of water back to her.

She swallows and I pray to God. Traffic starts moving again and I find the entrance to the LA Zoo. I frantically honk my horn, seeing Bethanne and Lynn caught up in a conversation of smiles. I call them over, then turn to Jani. "Get out now! Go with them and I'll find parking." Jani's bawling. I know she's upset because she never cries, but I can't comfort her this time. I'm too beaten down.

Bethanne and Lynn come over to the car and I burst into heavy tears. "I can't take her with me. I'm done." They look at me with sympathetic eyes as Lynn drops the blue gift bag next to Bodhi's car seat. There's no parking and I'm getting tired and I'm getting further frustrated driving in circles around this massive zoo parking lot. I can't stop crying. At least Bodhi's asleep.

My cell rings again. It's Bethanne.

"I can't find parking," I wail.

"Lynn and I have Jani. We're taking the kids to Shane's Inspiration. You'll find parking there."

"I have to call Dr. Howe. The Risperdal isn't working."

"Just take a break and we'll watch Jani for you."

"Thank you." Between the hormones, the exhaustion, and everything that's been happening, I am weeping so hard that I can't see the road I'm driving on anymore. I'm glad it's practically next door.

*   *   *

Through a cloud of tears, I drive slowly up the hill to Shane's Inspiration, a wheelchair accessible playground that allows kids who are blind, deaf, and wheelchair-bound to experience the same joys other kids do when they go to the park. Bodhi is still sleeping, so I pull over to a shady tree across from the park, page Dr. Howe, and just cry a river. Dr. Howe calls me back. "The Risperdal is not working," I tell her. "We were driving to the zoo and she tried to put the car into neutral *while I was driving on the 134.*"

"You need to take her to the hospital," Dr. Howe says, "I'm thinking she may have a Mood Disorder. I can call ahead and get you a Direct Admit at BHC Alhambra."

"What about UCLA?"

"If you can get in there, that would be great."

"Okay, let me call Michael." I hang up the phone and look back at Bodhi, still sleeping. I have no idea how long Lynn and Bethanne will be able to look after Jani along with their own kids. *I don't know what's wrong with me. Why can't I do this?*

I call Michael at work. "I need you to meet me at the zoo. I mean, Shane's Inspiration. We were supposed to go to the zoo, but we ended up here instead."

"What's going on?" Michael cool, calm, and collected tone makes me feel even more like a basket case.

"Jani had another episode. Bodhi was crying and she just flipped. She tried to put the car into neutral while I was driving and I just can't do this anymore." I know I'm babbling but I can't stop myself. "We need to take her to UCLA. I called Dr. Howe and she thinks it's a good idea."

"Okay, I'm coming."

"Good because I can't talk anymore." I hang up the phone and just breathe, like Michi always tells me to do. A few minutes later, I call Bethanne. "How's she doing?"

"She's doing… okay… at the moment. She threw a hissy fit earlier, throwing sand at everyone because she wanted to swing when it wasn't her turn and tried to push some other kids off."

"Lynn's girls?"

"No. They were off somewhere else. This was a kid I didn't know."

"Michael's coming and we're going to take her to UCLA."

"I think that's a good idea."

My heart skips a beat. Even when other moms were talking about Asperger's, Bethanne has always thought Jani's problem was our lack of discipline. "You think that's a good idea?"

"Yeah, I do." I wipe my wet eyes. "They'll know more about this," Bethanne speaks with conviction. One thing about Bethanne is that whether I want to hear it, or not, she tells it like it is, which makes me trust her opinion.

Michael shows up and we hug. Thank God I have him. He's my rock. I don't know what I would do without him. "So, it's been that bad, huh?" Michael looks directly at Bethanne, distrusting my intuition. *After all, how 'with it' am I anyway? I just gave birth a few weeks ago.*

"Yeah, I think you should go to UCLA," Bethanne says, her voice low. I know Michael hearing her say that we should take her to UCLA is shocking to his ears as well. Usually, she just says we need to be stricter. "You can't control her in the car. As much as you drive on the freeways, that's way too dangerous to ignore. UCLA is the best place to go. If you were back east, I'd say Johns Hopkins."

It would take a year and two hospital stays before UCLA finally admitted Jani. In that time, she would stay at both BHC Alhambra and the Loma Linda university hospital more than two hours from our home.

PART TWO

CHAPTER 10

THERE ARE PLACES FOR KIDS LIKE HER

March 14th, 2008

It's 10 pm when the pounding at the door starts. "Are you the parents of January Schofield?" A neatly dressed Hispanic man of small stature stands between two buff sheriffs' deputies. "I'm from DCFS, the Department of Child & Family Services." He flashes his badge. "May we talk with you?" He says this as if we have a choice.

"Yes," I say, my breathing shallow. Honey won't stop barking and looks like she is about to lunge but Michael keeps her close to him.

"There's been an allegation. We'll need to talk to both of you."

"That's fine," Michael says. "I just have to take our dog down to the garage."

"You're not going to run, are you?" Sheriff One asks.

"No," Michael says firmly. "It's just that our dog is territorial."

"Okay," Mr. CPS nods, eyeing Sheriff Two. I just bathed Bodhi and there is an uncomfortable silence as I continue drying him off. Michael returns quickly and their interrogation continues.

"I need to talk to you, Ma'am. In private," Mr. CPS tells me as they scan Michael. All eyes are fixed on me as I place Bodhi into Michael's arms and lead Mr. CPS in our bedroom. "You can sit there." He points to our bed where I sit as he stands looking down at me, ready to read the document before him. I listen intently as he begins. "There's been an accusation against your husband when he was giving your daughter a bath."

"Oh, my God! Michael does give her baths. So do I? We both take turns and wash her inside the tub."

Mr. CPS studies my face, awaiting more details. "Do you want me to go on?"

"Yes." Shockwaves ride up my throat. *Had she been molested?! Maybe she's not really bipolar at all!* "So, what did she say?"

"It says here that your daughter said, and I quote, 'When Daddy puts his finger up my pussy...my kitty cat goes meow.' "

My heart races a million miles per minute before taking a U-turn. "Wait a minute. Jani doesn't talk like that? That's street-talk. Jani's an intellectual."

"I know," his voice sympathetic, "because I already went out to BHC Alhambra and spoke with her. She said Mommy wipes her 50 percent of the time and Daddy wipes her the other 50 percent of the time. Even in the middle of delusions of 400 the Cat going under her bed, she told me this never happened."

It feels like your doctor saying "you have cancer" then recanting with "Ha! Ha! Just kidding!" I'm still rattled. "Well, then, what's going on? We put her in the hospital to get better!" I'm crying.

"Someone *said* 'she' said this and we're required by law to investigate. But here's what we have to do now," he continues. "I have to question him too, in case he confesses to something."

"Okay," I comply, just going through the motions. I don't have time to think. I walk out of the room with my head down, avoiding eye contact with Michael as I take Bodhi from his arms. Michael is led into the bedroom as I fall into the rocking chair, trying to pretend that two sheriff deputies are not hovering over me.

"What?! NO!!!" I hear Michael scream through the door. I am

reinvigorated, my heart still racing, tears gushing. I can't stop them. I can only wipe them away as quickly as they come. Michael and I are a team. It hurts to see him go through this but I can't bear thinking something like this might have happened to Jani.

"I'm really sorry," Mr. CPS tells us as we gather around the kitchen table filling out paperwork as the deputies relax their stance.

"So what am I supposed to do now?" Michael asks. "Not see my daughter?"

"No, you can still see her, but neither one of you can give her a bath or shower until April 14th, when the investigation closes. I'm really sorry." April 14th is our 8th anniversary.

They all leave but Michael and I are not the same. We are both shivering from the experience. I even feel uneasy laying next to him as he sleeps, his breathing heavier than usual. The seed of distrust has been planted and part of me is too scared for sleep. Did he really do something to Jani to make her the way she is? If he did then how could I lay next to him? *But then Jani was always different.* I HATE feeling this way, but I can't comfort or even touch him in this moment. I don't know where to put myself. I have to get Jani alone and ask her. Just to be sure.

*   *   *

The next evening, I get a moment to sneak in a private conversation with Jani. "I need to ask you something." She's eating the fried rice we bought her for dinner while I try to find the right way to bring this up. I don't have much time. Michael will be strolling in with Bodhi soon. "Did Daddy ever touch you, inappropriately?" From the earliest age, we've talked about this so she knows that no one is allowed to touch her private parts.

"Well, in the bath, when he was wiping me...one time it hurt."

"Was it with a washrag or his finger?"

"A washrag."

"Do you know what I'm asking you?" I have to move quickly with my questioning, but I need to hear my daughter say that nothing happened.

"Yes. I know what you're asking me."

"Did he ever touch you inappropriately?"

"No. He never did that." I sigh in relief at her reply as Michael strolls in with Bodhi. I feel like I betrayed him, but the Mother in me just couldn't shake this off. I hate this. I hate all of this!!!

Winter 2009

I'm running up the stairs with Bodhi in my arms. He's fifteen months old and should be walking by now. Jani was walking by eleven months, but he's such a warm, comforting generator in my arms that I don't force it. Besides, I've heard that lots of kids take even longer to start walking. Jani just happened to exceed all the milestones (except potty training). But then, what does all that mean now, anyway?

I'm practically out of breath by the time I reach the second floor, just in time for another visit from the Department of Child and Family Services (DCFS), otherwise known as Child Protective Services, or CPS. The social worker, Marla, called Michael earlier to notify us she'd be coming so we wouldn't be surprised this time.

"You probably know why I'm here," she relaxes her posture, holding her clipboard like we're old friends.

"Yeah." I put Bodhi down in his playpen so I can stand next to Michael as a united front. "But you do know that Jani is back in the hospital." My breath is still a bit heavy, after carrying Bodhi up those two flights of stairs.

"I know. I've been out to see her," she smiles then tags on a bit of humor. "She attacked me."

"That's Jani," I spontaneously giggle, trying to make light of the situation.

"I've already spoken with your husband," she gestures over to Michael, "about the report we received from a social worker."

"I was at a baby shower with Bodhi," I say, pointedly. "I don't really know what is going on."

She nods, looking over her paperwork. "He's being accused of 'abandonment and neglect'." I feel myself slipping out of my body. *Why is this happening?*

"Jani wanted to take Honey to the dog park," Michael starts explaining. "Central Bark, right by Central Park. At the last minute, she tells me that she doesn't want to go because she's afraid she'll hit the dogs if they jump on her, so I just let her play by herself in the sand park. I know I did a really stupid thing."

"Yes, you did," Marla agrees. "But I love dogs and I know the layout of the park." Her tone softens, "I know you didn't abandon her." We look at each other and sigh, relieved that we're not in trouble, but she's still staring at us like we're missing some other point she's trying to make. "You realize this will keep happening."

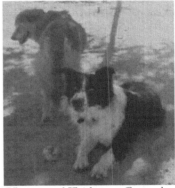

Honey and Friday at Central Bark.

"What do you mean, keep happening?" *Now I'm lost.*

"When you have a mentally ill child," she lifts her head up, trying to find the right words, "This is just what happens. People who don't understand the situation, *even other social workers,* call us."

"So what do we do? Are there any services?" I'm suddenly not so sure about this visit.

She shakes her head, apathetically. "Have you looked into residential treatment centers? There are places for kids like her."

"Our social worker at UCLA is trying to find one," Michael says, "but most of them don't take kids her age and the others are out of state."

"So what do we do now?" I question her.

"The most important thing you have to do now is..." she looks over at Bodhi chewing on a toy in his playpen "is keep *him* safe.

He's a toddler. He can't protect himself. Since she's in the hospital now, it's not an issue, but when she gets out, it will be. She's an immediate threat to his safety." She's so matter-of-fact about it.

My heart pounds, my voice shaking. "One of the problems we have now is that Jani leaves her bedroom door open. When Bodhi crawls in there and chews on her toys, it infuriates her." I turn to Michael for what to say next. He always has the answer, but this time he's ghostly white. *He doesn't know what to do.* "So this is because of Bodhi's age?" I ask.

"Your family is considered a high-risk case."

I channel Michi, and stand upright, maintaining good posture like a firmly rooted tree in the ground, a Bodhi Tree. "So, how old does Bodhi have to be in order for us *not* to be considered high-risk?"

She pauses for a moment, then flips her short strawberry blonde hair to the side. "Five."

I take in a deep breath then exhale. "Okay."

"I know this is a tough decision to make." She heads to the door, "but you have my number."

We watch her walk out in silence. Neither one of us can speak, but we both know what just happened. We've been given a choice. Do we keep Jani and lose Bodhi, or do we keep Bodhi and lose Jani?

*   *   *

I'm on Facebook, chatting with my friends when Michael calls. I hear the windblast through his cell phone so I know he's smoking, flicking ashes out the car window.

"Here's what we need to do," he starts off. I knew Michael would find an answer. He's a genius! I'm so glad I have him. "I will keep Jani here with me and we can send you and Bodhi back to your parents in the Bay Area." He has always been better with Jani than I have. He's more on her level. He keeps her brain occupied. I can't keep up with her but for some reason, I just can't do this.

"Huh?" I gulp a whimper down my throat.

"Look. I've figured it out. I'll fly up with Jani every weekend."

"But what about me?! She's my daughter too!"

"Yes, but you know how bonded she is to me. I can go back to teaching her every day and we won't have to worry about Bodhi's safety. He'll grow up in a better environment than we can give him now. He still has a chance."

"No," I tell him, abruptly. These days, tears pour out of me so fast and furious that I'm submerged under my own tidal wave.

"This is our only answer. If Jani hurts Bodhi, you know she'd never forgive herself. We'd lose both of them."

"You're right," I bite down on my lower lip. "But this can't be our only answer." Since I was laid off a few months ago, I can't even claim my job is keeping me here.

"It is. Unless you've got a better one?"

"Let's talk more when you get home," I say. The wave's impact passes over me and I rise up for air.

"Okay," he says and I release the call. There is no way I can do what he wants me to do. What will Jani think when she's older? That I chose her brother over her? Will Michael even know his son? Will Bodhi know his father? *Please, God, help me here…I'm begging!*

I turn back to my Facebook page where I've been updating details all night. I tell them Michael's idea and read the comments that come after.

My friend Irene, who used to drive me to youth group when we were in high school, is praying for me. Then there's Bethanne. She posts, "You could rent a duplex. That way, you're together, but keep the kids separate." *I'm liking this idea.* "But where?" I reply.

"They're hard to find," she posts back. "But search the Internet. The main thing is keeping them separated." *Oh, how I wish she hadn't moved back east last year.*

Then, it comes to me. "What if…and I know this is going to sound crazy," I type, but lose control of my fingers pressing the keyboard buttons fast and furious, "we move out of our two-bedroom apartment and into two one-bedrooms?" I type faster.

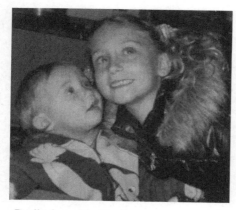

Bodhi loves his big sister.

"The kids would stay in the same place. Michael and I would switch off, like Jani's staff do at UCLA?"

Comments pour in and I can't scroll through them fast enough. Then my new support group friend posts. "We were going to rent the house next to us for the same reason." Maybe this idea isn't so outlandish?

I call Michael back right away and tell him my epiphany. "If it's meant to be then it will work. Talk to the manager tomorrow." She's always liked him.

"I will," Michael assures me. The very next day the apartment manager tells us that she has two one-bedrooms right across the parking lot from each other. *It was meant to be.*

CHAPTER 11

DON'T TALK TO STRANGERS

Summer 2009

Dinner time is at Bodhi's apartment. All the sharp utensils are kept high in the cupboards, just in case Jani goes into a violent episode where the nearest object becomes a weapon. When that happens, whoever her staff is immediately takes her out of Bodhi's apartment. The less madness he experiences, the better off he'll be. He deserves as much of a normal life as we can give him.

Tonight, the television plays in the background and to the outside world, we could appear to be a normal family having dinner together. "This is good," Michael says, nodding down at the salmon he prepared for himself.

"You're a great cook," I compliment him. "Your pasta primavera is still my favorite, better than any restaurant."

Jani is vegetarian but, unlike me, she won't even eat chicken or turkey on odd occasions. Bodhi has already shown us that he's a meat eater so Michael cuts off a piece of salmon for him to chew on while Jani and I eat our rice and we all share French fries. Bodhi finishes his meal before the rest of us and crawls under the table.

I stop for a moment, just to enjoy the calm with Michael. "Remember, when you and Jani came up with that restaurant idea? What was the name of it?"

"Oh yeah," Michael looks up. "Saddle Pigs! Remember that Jani?"

She doesn't answer, but instead looks up from her rice plate and lets out a piercing scream. "He's got my feet!" *Dammit!* Dinner time is over.

"Jani, stop it!" Michael yells at her and I feel his desperation. Whenever we get a just little peace we end up craving more, like a drug we can't get enough of. We're slowly making progress keeping her psychosis at bay by minimizing her stress, but at the same time, we have to give Bodhi a safe place to explore his environment so he doesn't grow up afraid of his sister. He needs to love Jani because eventually, he will be the one looking after her when we're gone.

"This is typical sibling behavior," I tell him. "I would do anything to get my older brother to play with me. The problem is that you grew up as an only child. He's just being mischievous, but it's getting late so we better go."

Bodhi giggles, still tugging at Jani's feet. She gives in to a healthy laugh then catches herself and yanks her foot away. "See, he's just trying to play with you." Michael is pleading with her, desperate for just a little more peace, but at least we made it through dinner. When Jani's schizophrenia was at its worst, we couldn't do that.

"Just..." Michael holds up his index finger, reaching for his cigarettes and lighter above the refrigerator, "give me a moment." He gives me this exasperated look before slipping through the sliding glass door so he can smoke in peace, just for a moment. I know this is hard for him, but it's hard for me too.

*   *   *

"Bodhi, NOOO!!!" Jani startles me. "That's mine!" Michael peeks in from the balcony. I can tell he feels safe out there. Free from our world.

"Jani, this is HIS apartment. He can play with whatever he wants," I continue to referee.

"How did he get my Pet Shop toy?"

"I don't know. Maybe you brought it in here?" I reach for Jani's toy but I'm too late. She grabs it out of his mouth and he starts bawling. "Give it back to him!"

"Fine! Keep it forever!" She throws it at him. "I don't want it anyway!"

He retaliates, pulling her straggly blonde ringlets and making her scream. "Bodhi! Let go of Jani's hair!" I know this is ordinary sibling rivalry, but they need to love each other. "Jani, we're going back to your apartment. NOW!"

Michael inhales an extra-long drag from his cigarette then smashes the butt into the ground before coming back in, a waft of smoke trailing behind him. "You can go now," he says, bluntly. Living apart has already taken its toll on us. Marriage is hard, and having a special needs child is hard, but living apart is just making it harder. This is probably why so many people have told me that when you have a child with special needs, the divorce rate is so much higher. But we're beating the odds! We just have to keep going. We've already made it for over a year now.

Tonight, it's my turn as Jani's staff. So many nights have run more smoothly than this one but it's like Michael always says, "One step forward, two steps back." I rush to gather all the things Jani and I might need for the next day then move over to kiss Bodhi goodnight. "Bye, Bodhi, I love you." I give him a tight squeeze. "I'll see you tomorrow."

"Just go." Michael shoos us off and we head downstairs, but by the time we reach the bottom, I hear Bodhi crying out and turn around to see the door fly open. Bodhi comes stumbling down the steps with Michael running after him. "Just go! He'll only keep crying for you."

I run over to Bodhi and pick him up, kissing him all over. "Jani and I will see you at school tomorrow morning. I love you," I linger.

"Come on, Mommy." Jani is pulling me toward her apartment.

"We'll be okay. Just go," Michael says, waving me off again.

"You're my staff tonight," Jani perks up.

"Yes." My head and heart hurt, still conflicted about whether or not we made the right decision. I turn to Jani. "What do you want to do before bed?"

"Hmmm. Let's play Chutes and Ladders in Mandarin," she tells me like we're having a slumber party.

"You are a genius!" My mind flashes back to what I'd always believed before her schizophrenia became my new reality. I'd still like to pretend it doesn't exist.

"So are you, Mommy."

"No, you get that from Daddy."

"Yeah, but you're the one who came up with the two apartments," she pats me on the back, giving me an indescribable feeling of euphoria. *Everything we've gone through is worth it.*

When we get up to her apartment I spread out the game mat with Chutes and Ladders and we roll the dice to count in Mandarin as they climb up ladders and slide down chutes. It's nice being able to give Jani my undivided attention, but I can't stop thinking about Bodhi. Ten minutes later, Jani is bored with the game. "I'm ready to read now, Mommy."

"Okay, but you need to take your meds." She follows me to a cupboard we turned into our own little pharmacy, high out of reach. I bring down each medication, making sure to look at every label. She's on so many pills now, but they're working. Each time I have to remind myself why I'm giving her these pills in the first place.

*   *   *

It's been another rough night so I read to Jani, then wait a few moments until I hear her delicate snore. Once I am sure she's asleep, I quietly slip out from underneath the covers and tiptoe into the living room to call Michael. When he answers I hear screaming in the background.

"Jani's asleep. How's Bodhi doing?"

"Not good. And I haven't had a cigarette in over two hours."

"Hmmm."

"What?!" Michael's anger penetrates through my cell.

"I'm just thinking of what we can do."

"Can you maybe come over for a minute? You said Jani's sleeping." The desperation in Michael's voice scares me. The arrangement is keeping Bodhi safe, but Michael and I are always on call. When we were together, we were never really alone. Now we are, and it's exhausting. I miss Michael and I being a team, but it's worth it to keep my babies safe and my family (mostly) together.

"I have a better idea. Let's meet in the middle of the parking lot and trade places."

"But what about Jani?" He hesitates.

"She'll understand." *I hope.* After years of Michael always being the one with the solution, it's nice to finally be the problem solver, at least sometimes. I hold onto my phone as I walk out to meet him, carefully watching my steps across the dark parking lot. When I reach the island, Bodhi's arms are outstretched, waiting for me to take him.

"You got him?" Michael seems so relieved.

"Yes." I snuggle him into my chest then carry him up to his apartment as Michael slowly climbs the stairs from Bodhi to Jani. The apartments are close enough to see, but not to touch or hear each other. I bring Bodhi to the rocking chair and cuddle him until he falls asleep in my arms. I know this can't go on forever. I just have to find the right balance between both kids' needs so we can make it through another day.

*   *   *

The next morning the phone rings and I automatically use my pet name for Michael. "Bo?" It's only when we're angry at each other that we 'drop the Bo.'

"Mommy?"

"Jani?" I take a moment to process the shock of hearing my five-year-old using her dad's phone that even I can't operate.

"Where are you, Mommy?"

"In Bodhi's apartment. He was having a hard time sleeping so Daddy and I switched last night." It's my only alibi, but it's the truth. "Is Daddy still sleeping?"

"Yeah."

"What time is it?" Silence. Even though Jani knows how to use Michael's phone, she still has a hard time communicating over it. My guess is that whatever invades her mind makes it difficult, especially since she hasn't had her morning meds. I repeat the question. "Jani, do you know what time it is?"

"7:04."

"What?! Daddy's gotta get up! He'll be late for work." I panic.

"Can I come over there?"

"Yes," I tell her. "But wait! I have an idea. I need you to get a cup and fill it with water. Then I want you to pour it on Daddy. That'll get him up." I smile to myself. "Can you do that?"

"Alright," she agrees, sharing a bit of my thrill.

"Just bring the phone with you so I can hear everything."

"Okay." The phone hits the counter as the cupboard doors bang around and the faucet runs.

"Do you have the cup of water?" I speak louder into the phone.

"Yep!" She sounds excited to follow through on this mission. Seconds later, a splashing waterfall spills through my cell.

"AHHH!!! What are you doing?!"

"Mommy told me to splash water on you to wake you up."

"Are you awake?!" I am yelling into the phone so he hears me.

"Yes...yes. I'm awake," Michael groans.

"Good, because you're going to be late for work. Can you get Jani ready and send her across the parking lot?"

"Yeah," he yawns. This isn't the first time Jani's come over while I've been Bodhi's staff. Michael has a hard time getting up in the morning to teach English classes at Cal State Northridge. He teaches online classes at night but mostly it's his chronic depression, which has only gotten worse over time. The kids are managing, but our marriage is suffering.

I go out to the balcony of Bodhi's apartment and wave to Michael across the way. He's in his boxer shorts puffing on his cigarette. We both watch Jani run down the stairs. I'm so proud of her. She looks both ways in the parking lot, even stopping at the island to make sure it's safe to cross over to the other side.

"Good girl!" I say, losing sight of her, then hearing hard footsteps pound up to the third floor.

She bursts through the door, "Is Bodhi up yet?"

"I'm getting him up right now."

"What can I do?" she whines.

"I don't know. I've got Nick Jr. on so you can watch Dora." Jani sits in front of the TV, moping, while I go back into Bodhi's room and pick him up as he comes awake, all smiles. I bring him into the bathroom so I can get bathed and dressed.

"We're ready, Jani!" I call out to her, holding Bodhi in my arms. No answer, but the TV is still on. "Jani?" My body tenses. This isn't a big apartment so I know within seconds that she's not here. *Dammit! If only Michael would just get up on time. I can't do two kids by myself!*

"Jani!" I set Bodhi down in his playpen and call out into the hallway of the complex.

A few seconds go by before I hear what I'd taught her to say at eighteen-months-old. "I'm right here!" She's walking alongside a young woman wearing a power suit, ready to take on whatever world she's living in because it's certainly isn't ours.

"She knocked on my door asking if I had any dogs or cats. I don't, but I told her that she shouldn't knock on strangers' doors." Her meds. I forgot to give Jani her meds.

"Thank you," I say, not having the will or energy to explain.

"You're welcome," she smiles then looks down sweetly at Jani. "Remember, don't talk to strangers."

"I won't," Jani replies, as the woman re-adjusts the computer bag on her shoulder and heads down to her car.

"What's going on?!" Michael pants, sprinting across the parking lot in his dress shirt and pants. "I heard you screaming for Jani."

"You really have to start waking up on time!"

"I know. I know." He brushes me off. It's not the first time he's heard it.

"I can't get Bodhi ready and watch Jani. She just left the apartment and knocked on a stranger's door asking if she had a dog or cat."

Michael sighs. Jani has done this before. It's typical of someone with schizophrenia. They get lost in their other world and Michael knows this. "Where's Bodhi? I've gotta drop him off at Kinder-Care."

"He's still in the apartment."

"You left him there?" He stands in judgment as I linger in the hallway. "Here you are chastising me and you're not exactly Mother Theresa yourself." *He's got me there.*

Bodhi is crying in his playpen when I go over to pick him up. He sticks to me like glue. "Do you want a pink donut?" Michael knows the right line to feed him.

"Yes." Bodhi blinks away a final tear and holds his little arms out for his daddy.

CHAPTER 12

PINK DONUT

Fall 2010

"I want to go to KinderCare and see Bodhi," Jani begs me. At her last IEP, we made it so that she could do "Home Hospital" on the school's site, but after all the other kids went home. That way if she goes into an episode, the other kids won't be at risk of getting hurt. We hope this will make it easier for her to eventually transition into a special education class.

"Remember, management told us we're not allowed to come in until 11 am, at the earliest." We already did breakfast at Western Bagel and reading at Barnes & Noble. "What about Chuck E. Cheese?"

"Okay," Jani agrees and we play there for a while. Jani always climbs up the play structure and crawls through the tunnel. She sits at the top, looking out at the world like a wild animal trapped in a cage. It's disheartening, watching all these new moms with their toddlers grouped together. That used to be us. Before everyone else started preschool and then kindergarten. Before Jani's hallucinations got so bad. Before Michael and I stopped being "mommy and daddy" and started being staff.

When we finally get to KinderCare, the kids are at recess and Jani runs out to join them. "Come over here, Bodhi! Let's go down the slide together." I sit on the benches next to the teacher and her aides. The sky is bright blue and the air is fresh. It's nice to see Jani actually being the big sister I'd always envisioned. Unfortunately, Bodhi doesn't seem to hear her. He's just spinning around in circles alone on the grass.

After recess, Jani and I give the teacher and her aides a break by serving the kids' their lunch. Some bang their blue plastic plates on the table, creating a drum circle, but not my Bodhi. He patiently waits for his sister to serve him his hamburger and mashed potatoes while I pour milk into their tiny plastic cups.

"Anyone want ketchup or mustard?" Jani holds up the bottles. Most of the kids' arms fly up. Jani relishes this part of her day and she's so good at it. I bring the bottles around, squirting the condiments on the kids' plates. "Finish your hamburgers," Jani firmly instructs the children even though she's a vegetarian and won't eat them. She hands a second serving to Bodhi, who made short work of his food. "Here you go, Bodhi." She places a second hamburger on his plate.

Michael comes to KinderCare after he finishes teaching and helps with clean-up. Bodhi doesn't nap anymore, which reminds me of Jani at his age, but we prepare a cot for him anyway, should he ever change his mind. An aide puts his favorite Cars blanket over him. Someone left it behind and they've given it to him for keeps.

We continue clearing the table. Bodhi isn't sleeping, which could be why the little blonde girl beside him is trying to start up a conversation. He looks at her, but then his eyes wander up to the ceiling. "Pink Donut!" His hand reaches up in the air and the little girl mimics him. Now they're both reaching up in the air, but Bodhi is getting angry. "I want it!" The little girl seems confused. "Pink Donut!" Bodhi grasps at the air again, his eyes following the phantom donut as he gets off the cot and chases it around the classroom.

"Did you get him a pink donut this morning?" I ask Michael.

"Yes. I always do that."

I call out, "Bodhi, you get a pink donut at the donut shop." He doesn't answer me, still preoccupied with the flying donut.

"There's no pink donut," Jani giggles. "He's schizophrenic." This jars me a bit, but I know Bodhi's already been diagnosed with Pervasive Development Disorder, a mild form of autism, so I can't say the thought hasn't crossed my mind, especially since his current behaviorist, Carrie, has seen him hallucinate. But it doesn't matter. Doctors wouldn't do anything for him at this point anyway. He's still years too young.

*   *   *

Bodhi can't continue at KinderCare. He's falling too far behind the other kids developmentally. However, he is entitled to free enrollment at our school district's autism preschool. We know he's smart because he follows directions. He understands everything but doesn't talk much and seems to go in and out of our world.

"There's Bodhi!" Jani claps like she's watching her favorite TV show when his preschool lets out at 11 am. Michael's off work so the three of us are here to pick him up. "What's he doing in the parking lot?!" Jani giggles. "That's silly."

My head spins, trying to comprehend what I'm seeing: Bodhi wandering aimlessly through the parking lot *alone!* "BODHI!" I call out, frantically running around the cars circling him. "What are you doing?! You could get hit by a car!" He seems disoriented and doesn't answer.

"I'll handle this!" Michael marches toward the aide who's still signing children back to their parents, but he's too slow to speak and I can't hold back. "You lost my son! He was walking around the parking lot in a daze!"

The aide guards the clipboard close to her chest. "I guess he escaped me."

"What's going on?" The teacher comes out and we rehash the incident. "I'm so sorry," she says, "That will never happen again."

"That's right, it won't happen again because he's not coming back to this classroom!" Michael is shouting. We are both furious. We call an emergency IEP for him. It's the first time I meet Aileen, the school psychologist, and I fall in love immediately. She seems to get Bodhi's issue from the start. We succeed in switching Bodhi to Ms. Tracie's class. We'd wanted Ms. Tracie in the first place because she works with Jani during Home Hospital.

This resolves the immediate problem but the underlying issue is not being addressed. So, I decide to make my suspicion known to this group of special needs' educators sitting around the conference table, especially Aileen, because she seems to be truly interested in what I have to say. "I know this may sound crazy, but please watch Bodhi closely. I think he might have schizophrenia, like Jani."

Aileen nods, her eyes taking it all in while the rest of the team sit around the table, probably thinking about what they're going to have for lunch.

CHAPTER 13

DON'T WORRY, BE HAPPY

Spring 2011

It's the end of the month, bills are due, and Michael has his "period." Dark, dilated pupils replace his normal salty blue eyes. "How are we going to pay rent?"

I knew I shouldn't have lingered with Jani after dinner tonight. It was just going so well with the kids together that I lost track of time. "I don't know," I try bringing him down to a whisper.

"We can't keep doing this," he starts to whisper-rage. Like couples with neuro-typical kids, we fight more and more about money as the kids get bigger and the bills grow with them.

"I really don't want to get into this now," I warn him.

"You haven't had an unemployment check in years," he says, like it was my fault I was laid off in September 2008. At the time, Jani was in and out of the hospital and I had to take Bodhi to work, hiding him in the studio, praying he wouldn't cry while I was on-air.

"Jani," I call out. "We're leaving now."

"We're going to have to move back in together." Michael won't stop.

"What about Jani. She's doing so well...."

"It's all her fault we're in this position in the first place!" This isn't like Michael, the old Michael. He always used to put Jani first and defend her from everyone else.

"Would you be quiet?!" I bring my voice down to a low, harsh whisper. "I hate it when you're like this." I turn to Jani, ready to cry for her. She loves Michael so much and when he says stuff like this in front of her, I just hate him. I will defend my kids against anyone, including their father.

"Do I look like I care?!" His rage intensifies. "Just LEAVE!" Michael pushes himself away from the table. I know this look. I've seen it before.

"I can't leave Bodhi with you when you're like this. I don't trust you!" Jani pulls me to her as I tell him this, wanting to leave, knowing Michael's mood shifts whenever the rent is due. But I don't go.

"You've *never* trusted me!" He's right. Ever since we got into a fight and he hit me in the back when Jani wasn't even two, I've never trusted his violent streak. Even though I struck back, punching him in the jaw (in self-defense, of course), I told him that he had to get help if we were to stay together. "Did you take your Lexapro?"

"I can't AFFORD my Lexapro!"

"Oh, God. Jani, we can't stay here but I can't leave Bodhi with him."

"It's okay, Mommy. Bodhi can sleep in my apartment," Jani offers. And these are the words I've been waiting to hear for years, but I never imagined them coming from a moment like this. I pick up Bodhi, still in his diaper, and we all walk out of his apartment and over to Jani's. I'm scared because I don't know where to go from here. I pray to God everything will work out and the old Michael will just come back. He usually does when I take control and prove that I don't need him. But I can never be sure and I really don't trust him, especially when he hasn't taken his Lexapro.

We're inside Jani's apartment. "Okay, Jani. Let's just get you in your bath and ready for bed."

"I'll get my pajamas. Just make sure he doesn't get into any of my toys," she says.

"I will," I tell her, as Bodhi rests quietly in my arms. We stand in one place because I have no idea what my next move will be.

"I can't do my hair," Jani shouts from the bathroom. I'm still afraid to put Bodhi down so I tell her to just wash her body for now and we can do her hair in the morning. She's satisfied with this so I call Michael and tell him to bring me more diapers. I'm keeping Bodhi here for the night.

A few minutes later, Michael appears. "I'm sorry," he says, full of regret. "I took my Lexapro. I hadn't had a cigarette in a while. I'm all right now. I can take Bodhi."

"Only if he wants to go."

"Bodhi, do you want to come with me? I'll read to you and we can play cars," He holds out his arms to Bodhi, his sugary sweetness making me cringe, but Bodhi goes willingly.

"I guess the positive here," I tell Michael, "is that now we know Jani's ready to move back into one apartment."

"Yeah," Michael sighs with an easy smile. It's been so long since I've seen that smile. I forgot what it looked like.

While Bodhi's at school the next day, we talk to the apartment manager about moving back together. "There is a two-bedroom available at the end of March, you just need the deposit. Do you want to take a look at it?" We all agree, and she takes the three of us on a golf cart ride over to our new place.

"Which bedroom do you want, Jani?" I ask.

"This one," she points to the left. Of course, it's the master bedroom with the attached bathroom, but we're fine with that. She's been through so much, this is the least we can do. The best part is that she's excited for all of us to be together again.

When Bodhi comes home from school, we bring his toys and lay them on the carpet so he can start getting used to the new place. All is good. We did it! We made it through two years of living apart to keep our family together.

*   *   *

I'm in Dr. Howe's office for Jani's appointment when she reads me Jani's latest test results. "Either she has an infection or something else is wrong." Because Jani takes Clozaril, (Clozapine), she is required to get weekly blood draws to monitor her white blood cell count. It's a medication of last resort but for the past couple years we haven't had any complications and it is working. The fear is that if her white blood cell count drops too low, her immune system will be compromised and she won't be able to fight off infections.

"Oh, my God!" This has been my biggest fear. The only medicine that works and now she's getting the side effects. "How low is it?" I brace myself.

"It's not low." Dr. Howe rolls her chair up to me so I can see the paper in her hands. "It's high." *Huh?* "See how it's usually between 10 and 12?" She flips through the previous weeks. "It's jumped to 17." I look over the test results as she swivels her chair toward Jani, who looks to be the stereotypical psychiatric patient, lying on the couch with her head on the pillow.

"How are you feeling?" Dr. Howe asks.

"Good," she answers.

"Does anything hurt?"

"No."

"We're going to move back into a two-bedroom apartment next month. Could anxiety be causing this?"

Dr. Howe shrugs. "It's possible."

"Jani, are you anxious about the move?" I ask her.

She sits up and looks directly at me. "Yeah," she admits. *Oh God, what are we going to do? We're all set to move in.* "Jani, what if we didn't move now? Do you think your anxiety would go down?" She nods, more disappointed in letting me down than worried about her own physical health. "Okay, then. We're not moving."

"Let's see what happens next week," Dr. Howe says. "It could just be a fluke, but what concerns me is that the jump is so high. Usually, when it's a fluke it only fluctuates a little, not this much."

When we get home I tell Michael the news and he agrees that we can't take a chance. So, we go back to the apartment manager and she lets us take back our notices to vacate the one-bedrooms.

Michael once again begs for money over his Facebook page and we're lucky that people who know our story donate enough for us to avoid litigation. He resents me when he has to beg for money, as if it's my fault I lost my job and we're broke.

The following week Jani's blood test comes back normal.

Chapter 14

Warrior Mom

October 2011

By fall 2011, Michael's complaining about money again. "I can't keep asking people to help us with the rent. Every time I do, people start telling us to move somewhere cheaper. They don't understand that Jani's health is at risk. I'm sick of it."

We're strolling Bodhi around the schoolyard while Jani's in her two-hour Home Hospital session. During the past couple of years, Jani has steadily improved, going from one to two hours of school with Ms. Tracie. She's even been able to do equine therapy at Carousel Ranch, a nonprofit that works with special needs kids, and volunteer with Michael at the Castaic Animal shelter.

"She wanted to move back together. I know she's ready. She even invited Bodhi for a sleepover. You know this is all because of her anxiety." I turn to him, excited by a new thought. "What if we set it up, but don't tell her about it until the last minute?"

"We'd be taking a risk." Michael considers this, watching some kids kicking around a ball. One boy gets knocked down then gets back up again. "But...it could work."

"It was the *prospect* of moving, not that actual move that caused her anxiety and we just made it worse by showing her the place. If we did it secretly and told her right before the move, then she wouldn't have a chance to get anxious."

We agree and our new move-in date is mid-October. This time, we've got a plan. I start bringing things over, careful to only take things from Bodhi's apartment. I don't want to give Jani any indication of what we're doing. The best part is that her blood draws are back to normal! As long as we keep her anxiety low, she should be okay. The doctors at UCLA told us a while back that she has a fragile mind and keeping her stress level at a minimum is crucial to her functioning in the outside world. A few days before the move, we're at Red Lobster when Michael drops the ball. "We still need to get the keys," he says.

"Are we moving?" Jani stares us down, not missing a beat.

I hesitate. Jani's keen sense of observation has always made it hard to hide anything from her, but I've always been honest with her because I want her to know that she can trust me. "Yes," I say, holding my breath.

"Don't worry, Jani. You'll do fine," Michael reassures her.

"I don't want to talk about," she gives us 'the hand' and goes back to eating her mac n' cheese. Michael gives me a 'this is it' look.

*   *   *

The AT&T guy crawls around on the carpet connecting cables while Bodhi sits in the middle of the living room playing with his cars. "I'm glad we made the move," Jani dances around our new place in her orange-flowered jumper.

"Me too," I smile, feeling like we've just ended one of the worst chapters in our lives. The only problem is that I can't seem to find our wedding rings. I put them in a safe place for the move, but now I can't remember where that safe place is? We look in my Grandma Freda's old jewelry box and other antiques I knew I was keeping, but for whatever reason, it's not there. Michael and I never see them again.

Jani and I go back to her apartment to get the red-eared slider turtles we rescued from the Castaic Animal Shelter. They wait in the bathtub until Michael and I lug their tank up to the new apartment. We make another trip out, bringing in more clothes, but by the time we get back, two statuesque women are standing in the middle of the living room. If not for the ID tags hanging from their necks, I'd think they were part of a thirty-something volleyball team. One is clearly the captain with thick brown hair flowing down her back. Her teammate wears a short brown wave.

"A call came in," the captain says. "It's not from a mandated reporter, but we have to take it seriously. You really have to be careful what you put up on Facebook." This tips me off that "Warrior Mom," an anti-psychiatry mother of two, probably called them. She is appalled at the medication we're giving Jani and the Benadryl I stupidly told her I was giving Bodhi to help him sleep at night.

"I know," I sigh. "He has autism and she has schizophrenia." I gesture over to Bodhi and Jani so they can check them out from head to toe.

"Is he getting any services?"

"Yes, he gets full ABA and some respite care."

The young women take their notes and ask for phone numbers of the people working with him, including Dr. Howe, his pediatrician, dentist, and behaviorists. "Is *she* getting any services?" the captain asks.

"No, she was denied because she's schizophrenic and not autistic."

"But she's autistic-like."

"Yes, that's what UCLA said too, but the regional center still denied us." I look them both straight in the eyes, the reporter in me taking over. "*This* is the problem with the mental health system in America today. There are barely any services, other than residential treatment centers where kids are getting abused, raped, even accidentally murdered."

"We know there are problems in the system," short-wave nods, like this upsets her as much as it does me.

"So, I'm speaking up about it."

"And you can do that," the captain takes over, "but you're taking a risk whenever you talk about your own kids over the internet. That's the reason we're here."

"Can you move this along," Michael sighs, irritated because he's being called yet again to help the cable guy set up the server for our internet connection in the new apartment.

"So you got the call..." I begin again.

"Are you giving Bodhi Benadryl at night?" she asks me, directly.

"Yes." The notetaking begins.

"How much are you giving him?"

"About a cap-full. Here, I'll show you." I get the Benadryl from the cupboard and demonstrate how much I put into Bodhi's juice at night.

"Have you talked about this with Dr. Howe?"

"Yes, and she says it's better than putting him on medication at this point." More writing. "Anything else?" I ask.

The captain's eyes veer over to Jani. "She's doing really well."

"She is. The only thing we could really use is help with her hygiene. She still can't take a shower by herself."

"Have you talked to the regional center about this?"

"Yes, but they say that she doesn't qualify."

"We can help you with that."

"Great!"

"Are you sure?" Michael's interest peaks.

"Yes, we work in the same office. All you have to do is fill out the paperwork and fax it over. We can make the call."

"I want to go to school now," Jani blurts out.

"Okay, just a few more minutes," I promise

The captain then turns to me, "Just make sure you don't say too much about your kids on the internet."

"Okay, I won't."

Now that we're all at ease I ask them if the call came from Warrior Mom and they grin. "All we can say is that it did not come from a mandated reporter."

"You know, we're around mandated reporters every single day, anyway."

"And that's what you need to keep doing. I may have more questions later," she says as they both get up to leave.

"That's fine. We're an open book."

"By the way," Michael stops them. "I have a book coming out in August and there are some things I'm not proud of, but they were a long time ago and I've been on Lexapro since then..."

"So, we may want to keep this case open if you think we're going to get more calls," the captain concludes.

Michael and I look at each other. "Let's do it," I say.

"And how are they getting along?" Their eyes dart between Jani and Bodhi, a subtle reminder that Bodhi is not yet five.

"They get along great," I shrug.

"She's okay with him?"

"Yeah," I say as we watch Bodhi in the middle of the living room talking to a few of his cars.

"Do you think he mimics her?"

"Sometimes he does, but he's not around her all the time."

She nods, taking another moment to study both of them. They may look neuro-typical on the outside, but they are clearly in their own separate worlds. Then Bodhi bursts out, throwing a car against the wall. "NO! I don't want it!"

My eyes turn to the captain. "I know he's diagnosed with autism, but just for the record, do you see anyone he's talking to?"

She flips her long hair to the side. "No, I don't."

"Neither do I."

*　　　*　　　*

We're at Bodhi's IEP and Aileen is reading quickly through Ms. Tracie's notes as though it's necessary nuisance. "So, Bodhi likes to play with his cars, has an imaginary friend, and enjoys circle time."

She flips over to the next page.

"Wait! Hold on here." I shake my head, forcing her to backtrack to the 'imaginary friend' part.

Aileen looks at me and downplays my concerns. "You know this can be completely normal. He's almost four and a lot of kids have imaginary friends."

"The problem I'm having is that I heard the same thing from the Rinaldi Adult School when Jani and I were in a Mommy & Me preschool." I look to Ms. Traci. "Who is this imaginary friend?"

"I'm not sure what his name is. Maybe Carlos? And he spaces out sometimes." The countdown has begun.

"I think its Carson," I tell her. "We've heard him mention the name before. Jani thinks it's because he like cars so much."

After the IEP, I contact Dr. Howe and she makes a separate appointment for Bodhi. She's already seen the video I took of him looking out of the window, pointing to something, then getting scared and screaming. He'd turn away and calm down for a few moments before it started again.

"You know," Dr. Howe says, seriously. "I'm not discounting the video you showed me." She tries to talk to him, but he's not saying anything right now. "Let's just keep an eye on him. That's all we can do at this point."

CHAPTER 15

A STARBUCK'S MOMENT

Late October 2011

These days, I rarely ever get a "Starbuck's Moment," but today I finally get the chance and I grab it. Lynn and I lost touch after Jani went into BHC Alhambra. UCLA wouldn't take her at that time and she was in there for three weeks. In the meantime, Lynn kept calling me for playdates with her girls, but Jani was hardly home and, truthfully, I was jealous that she and her daughters were moving on with their lives while we were stuck in a rut.

Ironically, it was Bodhi who reacquainted us. Last Mother's Day, Bodhi ran off across the grassy field at the Richard Rioux Park in Stevenson's Ranch. I suppose he was looking for a better variety of food because he attached himself to another family having a picnic, with blankets spread out across the lawn and a plentiful supply of snacks including hot dogs and hamburgers.

"I remember you. You're Lynn's mom," I smile and she smiles back as her grandkids play games around the picnic table. "Is Lynn here?"

"She should be back any minute."

It isn't long before Lynn arrives. Elizabeth and Corrine are the oldest of the grandkids. They immediately start throwing a football around with their dad and I'm practically crying. I wanted so badly to reconnect with her but I didn't know how. So many times, I wanted to make the call but I just couldn't do it. The guilt was overwhelming. The last day I'd seen Lynn was that awful day at the LA Zoo and Shane's Inspiration. And of all people to reunite us… Bodhi.

"Life hasn't been easy for us, either," Lynn tells me as we catch up in the coffee shop. "The girls mostly play with each other and then when it comes to having friends, there's always some issue, one likes the other more or some other girl drama."

"I remember when they were all three, eating ice cream at the Burbank Mall. It was after playing at Sweet Little Faces and you said that you wanted to just keep them this age forever."

"That was a nice time."

"But I didn't. I couldn't wait for Jani to grow up. I guess I was just having so many different experiences than you were, even then." She gives me a compassionate smile as she holds her coffee.

"Remember, we even traded kids once at the park. I pushed your girls on the swings, while you engaged with Jani. I remember Elizabeth and Corinne had a different energy. Not so intense." She nods. None of us at the time really knew what was going on. All we knew was that Jani was different from the other kids, which makes it comforting now because I can talk to her, no back-story needed.

My cell rings… "Uh-oh."

"Who is it?"

"The school." I close my eyes after seeing the number.

"Jani?"

"No…Bodhi." I hardly even notice I am whispering. "This is Susan." Lynn takes a concerned sip of her coffee while I process the new charge against my son. "Bodhi is out of control and biting. They want me to come pick him up now."

"I'm so sorry." Lynn looks pained.

"It's happening again," I tell her. "I can't believe this is happening again?!" My sadness turns to fear, then anger. "But I knew this time. I *told* them and they ignored me!"

"Do you want me to come with you?"

"Yes. Please," I break down.

Lynn and I get to the school just as the principal opens the door. She stands there like she's just seen the movie *Seed of Chucky* while Bodhi races down the ramp like a madman on speed. "He bit the aide." Her voice is fearfully stern. "We had to send her to get a tetanus shot."

"Good!" I walk up the ramp while Lynn observes my overreaction, followed by my tears. "I've been telling you this for months, but you didn't believe me. I guess *this* had to happen first for you to take me seriously!" The principal sighs, the expression on her face morphing from anger to sadness.

"Please, just do me a favor and write up a note. I will take it to Dr. Howe and then *she* will have a reason to prescribe the medication he clearly needs for his *schizophrenia*!" I hate that no one will say the word but they will stand in judgment of the actions that come from him going untreated.

"I will," she says sympathetically as Lynn helps me wrestle Bodhi into her Caravan. He's kicking and screaming but I sit with him, holding him protectively like a mother bear wrapping her arms around her cub. I'm amazed that Lynn drives steadily, looking back at us at every stop, yet maintaining her composure as Bodhi continues kicking the back of her seat.

* * *

"There's Pop Goes the Weasel!"

"Where's Pop Goes the Weasel?" Dr. Howe asks, Bodhi.

"Right there," he points up over her hutch then falls to the floor, laughing hysterically.

I hand her a note from the school describing the incident where he bit his aide. "It came out of nowhere. She needed a tetanus shot."

"We're going to put him on Risperdal."

"Okay," I nod, knowing that I can't say anything else because this is a process we have to go through. I think of it as a "game" we have to play. Sure, I suspect schizophrenia, but if Dr. Howe were to diagnose this so early in the process, she'd be in a lot of trouble. There are still psychiatrists and "Warrior Moms" who don't believe mental illness exists in children. So she has to play the game and so do we. Also, we'd have a lot harder time getting him services if he weren't diagnosed with autism.

*　　　*　　　*

"I scared!" Bodhi's been awake for a while now.

"What are you scared of?" I ask, hoping he'll give me a clue that I can run with here, but he doesn't. He just closes his eyes, hiding himself in my embrace. Some months ago, he startled me when we were sleeping. He sat up in the middle of the night, and said, "N is the 14th letter," then his head fell down on the pillow and he went back to sleep. I remember being so fascinated that as soon as he got up in the morning I asked him. "Bodhi, what's the 14th letter?"

"N."

Hmmm. "What's the 15th letter?"

"O."

"What's the 26th letter?"

A few seconds go by, then… "Z." WOW! He's numbered the alphabet and knows it to a "T," which is the 20th letter. In my entire life, I've never thought to do this. I wonder what else is going on in his mind. Clearly, he's smart and part of me is excited, but then there's the other part, the part that's scared for him.

Meanwhile, Jani has improved enough that we rework her IEP, praying to transition her smoothly from Home Hospital into her Special Ed classroom. First, we introduce her to physical education. It is less stressful and she'll get to meet the kids who would be in her class. Michael and I sit on eggshells watching the clock tick by in the school's office. Then, after a few days, it happens. She wants to follow the other kids back to their class. She connects with her teacher, Ms. Nelson, and it doesn't take long before she's able to do three and a half hours, a full morning, with her classmates. And then there are more benefits for Jani.

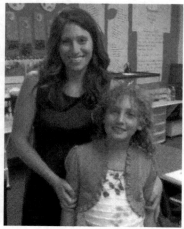

Jani's first school open house after transitioning from home hospital.

"Can we stop at Starbucks? Evan Miller drinks hot chocolate and he's ten. I'm ten, so I should drink hot chocolate too." Evan Miller is Jani's first schoolgirl crush. He is one of the reasons that Jani stays in class for so long, and I thank his mother.

"Sure, we can stop there." I smile at Jani. This is so cool. I feel like a normal mom bringing my two kids to Starbucks before school. Bodhi is still struggling in preschool, but they're not pressuring him in any way. So, it's basically just a nice three and a half hour break for me while both my kids are in school. After nearly a decade without any breaks, I'm in Heaven! I get to go shopping *by myself*!

On our way into Starbucks, I keep a strong hold on Bodhi's small hand. Jani's fast to order so I reach into my purse for a couple of dollars. "Put the change in the tip jar," I tell her, wanting her to be conscious of tipping as a nice gesture. She drops the change in and we walk over to the counter to wait while the barista makes her drink. Bodhi is getting restless, twirling around me, but I've got a solid grip on him. Jani stares at the barista, making sure everything is done to the last detail. Then... "AHH!" In a split second Bodhi escapes me and jets toward the door.

"Bodhi, come back here!" I look over at the heavy door he's trying to push open. There's no way he'll get through, but he does! I push through statues of people, past chairs and tables, running out of the coffee house. "BODHI!!!" A car comes out as Bodhi hits the street, but I catch him just in time, pulling him back to the sidewalk, holding him close while I squeeze his hand.

I know what's happening here. People probably think this is just a little boy running into the street. But, it goes way deeper than that. Whatever frightened him seems to have gone for the moment, but what was he running to? Or from?

Unfazed, Jani is sipping her hot chocolate as she comes out to meet us. No one would ever know what *she* went through–what we all went through–to get to this point. After dropping Jani off at school, I drive to Bodhi's school and park in the designated spot for kids with special needs and autism. It's a constant reminder that what we're going through is not normal. I walk Bodhi up to his classroom, feeling good seeing how happy he is in this moment, his aide taking him into her arms.

When I pick him up a few hours later, he stops short in the doorway. "I need to see Dr. Howe," he says like I'm his personal secretary. He's so serious and straightforward, just like Jani was when she knew she was slipping.

Why can't I be relieved that he has insight? The reality hits me. He was supposed to be Jani's savior, but now I fear for them both. What if I weren't here? No, I have to be here. This is a calling and God has chosen me to be their mother for a reason.

Bottling my tears, I take him back inside the classroom and wait for all the other kids to be signed out so I can talk to Ms. Tracie alone. She puts out some toys to occupy Bodhi. "How is he doing, Ms. Tracie? Really?"

"He's making it through," she says, solemnly.

"That's good. Any talk about the 'friend?'"

"Sometimes. He still spaces out a lot." I nod, keeping the cap on my tears. She looks at me, more like a friend this time. "But you knew it was more than autism." I nod and agree. *Yeah, I knew.*

CHAPTER 16

FOREVER IN DIAPERS

Spring 2013

Bodhi is sleeping one night on and one night off. And now, I've run out of diapers. Great. I suppose this is the perfect time to start potty-training him at night, but I hate to wake him up. Then again, he's not getting any younger, so it's either now or never.

I feel his pajama pants. He's dry! He must sense my presence because he slowly stretches out his little arms and legs. He comes awake and smiles at me.

"Bodhi," I ask him. "Are you wet or dry?" I always connect the words to what is happening with his body.

"Dry," he answers.

"Okay, let's go." I take his small hand in mine and move him quickly to the potty. I don't want to lose this opportunity. I pull his pajama pants down and lift up his shirt. "Three-two-one... blast off!" A stream of pee showers in and around the toilet with a fair portion making it in. I did it. I got him! "Good boy!"

*   *   *

I don't usually notice that I have eyelids until they're so heavy that I can no longer keep them open. Bodhi is in one of his bad sleep cycles. The problem with tonight is that he pulled an "all-nighter" last night and is still up for the second night in a row. Michael comes into my bedroom to tell me the "good news."

I look at the time. "It's past 1 am. You mean, he *never* went to sleep?"

"Nope."

"Okay." My body is heavy, ready to collapse underneath me, but I can't give in to it. Michael doesn't bother to change his own clothes, but simply takes off his jeans and rolls himself under the comforter on the carpet while Bodhi jumps in and around him like he just slept through a weekend that never existed. I give him Benadryl and lure him into the bath, but he still doesn't look tired, just a bit calmer. Instead, he jumps out of the bath and wanders around our apartment while I get him fresh pajamas and turn on cartoons.

He storms over to the refrigerator, eyeing the eggs. "Are you hungry?" It's the logical question, but logic has never been a big part of our lives.

Bodhi takes the eggs out and begins throwing them around. "I threw eggs!" He stares down at them, then back up at me, his eyes wide with shock.

I remain calm and try some logic. You never know. Maybe he really is 'severely autistic' and can't find the right words. "Do you want scrambled eggs?" He doesn't answer, but I get a pan out and make them anyway, preparing bacon and toast, one of his favorite meals.

He runs for the balcony and I turn to chase him but slip on the slimy eggs covering the floor. He's trying to open the door. It's locked pretty tight and his fine motor skills aren't that good–or, so I thought. Of course, he makes it outside. I block his move by the ledge and drag him back inside then quickly get the duct tape to lock the balcony door.

I'm not processing any of this, just reacting, but reminiscent tears fall anyway. He calms a little again. I think the Benadryl is kicking in. He's finally sitting in one spot, flipping through one of his books. "Bodhi, I made you scrambled eggs, toast, and bacon too." He comes over to look at the plate then swipes it off the table, making it splatter onto the carpet where Honey cleans up the mess.

I hate to do this, but I'm getting so frustrated that I go over to Michael and shake his comforter. Nothing. I shake it some more. Still nothing. Now, I'm really shaking it. "You have to get up!"

"Wha...wha...." He looks around and sees Bodhi. "He's still up?"

"Yes, and he's ready to go...somewhere? He hasn't gone down at all and I haven't gotten any sleep so you're going to have to get up." I hand him over to Michael. My patience is wearing thin, even with Michael. "We're going to have to take him to the hospital. His meds aren't working and you just go to sleep. I'm paging Dr. Howe."

"I'm not getting up now." Michael hands Bodhi back to me, but he is still flat on his back when Dr. Howe returns my page. I put the phone on speaker and bring it over to him.

"Did you try Benadryl and Melatonin?" she asks.

"Yes, we did," Michael comes awake because he is The Man. I hate myself for hating him even though he hasn't done anything wrong. We're both just so incredibly tired right now and it's tearing us apart.

"Then I don't know," she says.

"What about Thorazine?" I ask her, knowing that it's worked in the past to get him to sleep, but also knowing that I can't give it to him without a doctor's order.

"That's for emergencies," she says.

"He didn't sleep last night and he didn't nap during the day and he's up all night now!" I know it's not her fault, but I'm yelling into the phone.

"Did you try Ativan?"

"Not yet...."

"Try that first," she says, half-asleep, then hangs up.

A half hour passes and Bodhi's still running around. I get into the shower, splashing water all over my face, and come out to Michael. "The Ativan isn't working. I'm taking him to UCLA."

"Huh" is the only response I get from the body bag on the floor. I put Bodhi's shoes on and go through the motions. Why not? What else am I going to do in the middle of the night? I close the door thinking I can bring more clothes tomorrow anyway. *Oh yeah, this is tomorrow.*

"No!" I hear Michael coming out of the apartment but ignore him. He's only going to yell at me so I just keep walking down the steps toward the car. "They're not going to do anything! We just have to ride this out!" He's running after me in his t-shirt and boxers.

"I'm too tired to stay up all night again." I strap Bodhi into his car seat.

"So how are you going to make it there if you're so tired?"

Michael's right. I turn to face him. "Then page Dr. Howe again. She listens to you more than me." When he agrees, I take Bodhi out of his car seat and the three of us walk upstairs. Thank God Jani sleeps through the night now that she's on the right medication. Bodhi's not. "If she doesn't call back soon, I'm giving him a Thorazine."

"Fine," Michael says.

After waiting about 15 minutes I watch Michael wrap himself up in his navy comforter. "She's not calling back."

"I think she fell asleep," he mumbles.

"I'm giving him the Thorazine. Dr. Howe didn't say not to, just that we had to try Ativan first and we did," I tell him, mashing the 25-milligram pill and putting it into a small cup filled with juice. Michael groggily agrees and within twenty minutes, Bodhi's sound asleep.

*   *   *

Things have been escalating for months with Bodhi. Now, I'm

in the kitchen holding his arms against the floor so they don't find their way into his mouth. If I fail, he'll bite down so hard that he will leave bite marks on himself. I can't even get him to a standing position. I am trying to calm down our five-year-old son enough so I don't have to ask Michael for help. I think he's schizophrenic like Jani–she's said it herself–and that he needs to go inpatient at UCLA. We have to get Bodhi there before he hurts himself. The problem is that Michael disagrees. I'm dreading the inevitable confrontation but I can't wait anymore. "Michael, HE NEEDS TO GO TO UCLA!"

Michael is in Jani's room changing the turtle tank. This is not his favorite job. I'm yelling but he's either pretending not to hear me or tuning me out. He comes into the kitchen carrying the hose to drain the turtle tank. "Do you see what's happening here?" I beg him to take a hard look. I want him to see what is happening to his son. *It's so hard and it hurts so much, but how can he not see?*

"He'll calm down eventually." Michael is focused on the hose he's screwing into the faucet, draining the water from the tank. He isn't looking at his son much less listening to me.

"He's not! He's doing this about 25 times a day. I can't take it anymore!" Michael thinks I just want to dump Bodhi at UCLA so I can get a break. He sees Bodhi improve for a little while but he isn't here to see how quickly it all falls apart again. This is not normal and it's getting worse, not better.

Michael walks away, leaving me on the kitchen floor with Bodhi thrashing in my arms. "Deal with it! I'm not taking him!" He's so different this time than he was with Jani. We both are. Jani bonded so closely with Michael and I believed that he knew best for everything with her. I learned a lot with Jani and this time I trust myself more.

"Don't yell at me! Dr. Howe said he should go to UCLA to be tested for 'seizures,' remember?"

"Yes, but that's not what *you* want. You want him to go inpatient."

"Yes, but it doesn't matter what I want anyway. If you don't take him to be tested for 'seizures' *right now*, then I will."

"And how are you going to do that? You can't even get him calm enough to sit in the car!" Michael waves me off. *What a fucking asshole!* But he's right. I can't do anything in this moment. I just have to ride through this thrashing until he wears himself out then prepare for the next round. "I know you don't want to go through this again, but I can't keep living like this. It's the same as Jani. We're living on eggshells."

Michael grips the far edges of the turtle tank like he's about to fall in. "It's not the same as Jani."

"Fine! Then just take him to get tested for 'seizures' because he's suffering right now. Correll owes us hours anyway." Correll is one of our respite workers for Bodhi. She's in her 50s and even though she raised three boys, she, too, is finding it hard to keep Bodhi under control by herself.

"Oh-kay," he relents. "If it'll get you off my back, then I'll call Correll, but all we're doing is getting him tested for seizures. *I'm not* putting Bodhi inpatient."

*   *   *

Michael calls me from UCLA, in tears. "They want to admit him."

I'm in shock. "What? You just got to the hospital two hours ago." Whenever we dealt with Jani going inpatient we'd have to wait at least four hours before getting a psych consult and even more hours to find out if a bed was available.

"I know, I know, but they took one look at him and said it's not neurological. It's not seizures. It's psychiatric. They put us in...." He can barely get out the sentence and I'm straining to hear him.

"They put you in..." I prompt, holding the phone closer to my ear.

"They put us in the same room I was in with Jani that first day she came here." He's sobbing into the phone. Even though I was pushing for this, I didn't really believe it was actually going to happen. "He's not good. Correll and I are trying to keep him from hurting himself. We can't even get him to the bathroom. They had to put him back in diapers."

"They put him back in diapers?" I cry. We worked so hard to get him potty-trained. Sometimes it seems like my babies are forever in diapers.

"It's for his safety." Michael chokes on his words. "We couldn't even get him to the bathroom without him trying to hit himself on the wall of the urinal." It's during these moments that I forget how much I hate Michael sometimes. Now, I have to be the calm one.

"He just needs to get on the right meds," I tell Michael, but it's more for myself to hear. This can't really be happening. Bodhi's my baby. He's alright. He has to be alright, for Jani. And as much as I hate to admit it, for me.

CHAPTER 17

I ALMOST KILLED THE FISH

Spring 2013

Bodhi's on UCLA's observation unit so they can so they can keep a close watch on him in their highly-structured environment. "I called the hospital and so far he's doing well," Michael says, apathetically.

"That's what they always say. Then the next day, the story changes to 'he's doing a lot better *today* than he was *yesterday*.' We both know the game here." After all we've been through, starting it all over again, Michael sounds defeated, so I make the call. "Hi, this is Susan, Bodhi's Mom. I want to check in on a few things. First, does he have a one-to-one yet? When we visited him last night his arms and legs were covered with bruises."

"No," the nurse answers.

"What?!" This is the problem with knowing too much this time around. "He *needs* a one-to-one."

"We haven't seen anything that would constitute it."

"But he's got bruises up and down his arms and legs!"

"You have to talk to the doctor."

"Never mind. We'll be in later." I hang up and look to Michael for answers. "So once again, he has to really hurt himself first before they'll do anything."

"Pretty much." Michael still hasn't recovered from the sleepless nights or from Bodhi's intake this time.

*   *   *

"I miss Bodhi," Jani comes into the kitchen, still in her pajamas. It's so nice to have her sleeping through the night these days. She's older and her meds are working. I keep reminding myself of all the guilt and relief I felt when she was inpatient. Now Jani's very independent. She can do everything except take a shower by herself. But since the last CPS visit, we actually have help for this.

"Let's get you into the shower now."

"Isn't Yvette coming?" Michael asks.

"Yeah, but I can't remember when."

"That means I'll have to take a shower… again!" Jani says angrily, 'tween 'tude' on full display.

"Unless I can get her to come in the mornings," I throw my hands up, leading Jani into her bathroom then guiding her through the steps to wash her body. "You're doing amazing!" The only help she really needs is washing her hair, so I rinse it out for her.

"My eyes!" The slightest bit of soap or shampoo brings out that piercing scream. I hand her a dry washcloth and she smacks her face with it then hands it back to me. "I'm *soooooo* itchy!!!"

"I can put lotion on you."

"That won't help," she whines. I wish she'd just be able to do this by herself. I also wish that Yvette would come in the mornings to get Jani on a regular schedule. She needs to learn this by rote. I'm not expecting miracles here, just for her to get by in the world without having to rely on someone else to give her a shower.

My phone rings and I walk out to the kitchen. It's a 310 number so I know it's UCLA. "Is this Mrs. Schofield?"

"Yes. What's going on?"

"This is Doctor Allen, the pediatrician."

"Yes," I am relieved that Bodhi is finally being seen for all his bruises.

"I'm a little concerned about something."

"Well, you should be! He's got bruises up and down his entire body and he didn't have those going inpatient!"

"That's not what I'm concerned about." His voice is more serious than I'd expected. "He's got a big bump on his forehead."

"He didn't have *that* when he got there!"

"I know. He got it here, but he did pass the neurological exam. We'll keep an eye on it."

"He needs a one-to-one AT ALL TIMES!" I'm yelling again but it doesn't seem like they listen unless I'm yelling.

"I agree with you. I'm going to get the psychiatrist to call you back. I just wanted you to know what I'm doing on my end."

And there it is. He finally hurt himself enough to get the one-to-one he should've had in the first place. "Thank you." I am breathlessly bitter as I hang up and turn to Michael. "Well, he's finally getting a one-to-one. He somehow banged his forehead so hard they had to give him a neurological exam! Clearly, the medication is not working! How much more does he have to go through for them to see this?"

"I don't know," Michael says, softly, taking his turn being the calm one.

*   *   *

Yvette arrives by late afternoon, wiping beads of perspiration from her forehead. "I just finished my class. Is Jani ready for her shower?"

"Yeah, she's in her room." Seconds later, we hear Jani screaming as Yvette calls out for help. I open the door with Michael behind me to find Jani out of the bathroom, hitting and kicking Yvette in her bedroom. She hasn't done this in a long time.

"I almost killed the fish!" Yvette is holding her, but Jani is jamming her legs at the white dresser drawers holding her small pink and blue fish aquariums. We were told that Betas can kill each other if they are put in the same tank so we've kept them separated, but every so often I see their noses trying to touch each other through the glass like they want to be together. Now they have a shared experience. They both felt an earthquake rock their worlds.

"Jani, if you're getting too violent, you'll have to go to the hospital too."

"I want to go!"

"Is this because Bodhi's there?"

"No," Jani says, unconvincingly. "I almost killed the fish, so I have to go." Michael and I trade glances, both thinking the same thing. A break! For the first time since before she was born.

"If she goes," Yvette turns to me, "I need to know for my schedule." *Of course she does.* This is what's so tricky about mental illness. Just like a neuro-typical person, a mentally ill one can lie. In this case, Jani may not be truly psychotic, but she's definitely stressed. And it would be nice for Bodhi to have his big sister there to comfort him.

Michael makes the call to Dr. Hyde and he tells us to go through the emergency room.

*　　*　　*

It's been so long since Jani was last hospitalized but most of the faces are still the same. Gillian remembers Jani and Bodhi from the beginning. She comes out to the vestibule where we're waiting, like well-rested parents returning from a lengthy vacation, to ask how we are. The sight of her is a relief. Bodhi's known the staff here most of his life. "We're okay. How's he doing?"

"Ehh," she nods to the side. "He's been up and down most of the day." She waves us through the double doors. "But the cutest thing happened." She tears up. "When Jani came onto the unit, they were both so excited. They ran up to each other and hugged!" She puts her hand over her chest, as my eyes turn into automatic waterfalls. *I knew Jani didn't have to come here. She just wanted to make*

118

sure her baby brother was okay.

"I'm so glad," I wipe the tears from my nose and cheeks.

"She's helping, too," Gillian says as we walk onto the ward. "She's telling the nurses how to calm him down. That he likes to rock and spin in the chair…. Look who's here?"

Jani and Bodhi bound up to us, wearing the brightest expressions like they're at their favorite summer camp. A huge weight is lifted off my shoulders. I always thought that Bodhi was going to be Jani's savior and now it's reversed. My vision of the future is completely skewed. I have no idea who will be taking care of whom? Or, will they take care of each other?

On our way back to the car, Michael and I are childless. We pass all the same landmarks like CPK but this time we're not limited to going to a "kid" restaurant. Instead, we drive home and enjoy a nice quiet meal at El Torito.

A week later, Jani's released without any med changes but for the first time, she engaged in talk therapy. There was a time when she wasn't even able to concentrate on a conversation for a few minutes let alone talk to someone about her feelings. When Bodhi is released the following week, he's not much better than when he went in. I have a feeling this is just the beginning for him.

CHAPTER 18

WE'RE NOT PILL PUSHERS HERE

Summer 2013

Bodhi's preschool days are drawing to a close and we're touring the kindergarten for mild to moderate autistic kids in the same school. When we get to the actual classroom, the kids are not the same as Bodhi. They're quieter. They don't talk as much as "regular" kids, but they pay attention to the teacher, giving robotic answers that are well thought out and make sense. Bodhi is like this sometimes, but other times he's outward, rambunctious, even engaging.

"Do they come in this way?" Michael asks the vice principal.

"No," she laughs. "There's a lot of agitation at first but once they settle into the highly structured routine they do very well." Michael and I look at each other, knowing Bodhi likes other kids because he plays with them at the hospital, but also knowing that he's not like these kids.

I look over my shoulder, hearing the familiar computer suitcase rumbling over the cement. Aileen, the school psychologist, is leaving Bodhi's classroom. "How's he doing?" I ask her.

She gives a half-smile. "We're letting him do what he wants."

"Good. Whatever he can do is fine. We don't want to put any stress on him."

*   *   *

Either Michael or I need to be home with the behaviorist at all times and since Michael's out, it's my turn. At least while they are here I can take a bath by myself, as long as I'm on-call if there's any kind of emergency. Yvette is also Bodhi's behaviorist and she's working to get him to eat some fruit snacks. Whenever he stops eating and sleeping, it's a bad sign for what's to come.

I manage to make it through, feeling refreshed, dressed in my comfy pajamas when I walk out to see Yvette and Bodhi sitting at the kitchen table. She's charting Bodhi's progress when Jani walks by and pops one of his fruit snacks into her mouth. In a flash, Bodhi screams, flipping backward in his chair, his head and back striking the carpet. "Oh, my God!" I go to my knees over to him.

"Just calm down, mom," Yvette reminds me. *Oh, how I hate this. It's not her child!* It's easy for her to stay calm as we both look him over to see if he has any injuries.

"I didn't do anything," Jani defends herself. "I just took one fruit snack."

"No, you didn't do anything." I am crying again as I reassure Jani. "He's just not on the right medication!"

"It doesn't help that you're screaming." Yvette strong-eyes me.

"I know." I bring my over-reaction under control. "We're just lucky he fell on the carpet. It could have been a lot worse. Please write this down in your notes." She promises, but how can I *not* worry? It's like I'm living on the edge of an invisible cliff.

*   *   *

Back in 2009, I bumped into Dr. Hyde walking into the vestibule at UCLA. He was always in a hurry so I quickly asked him what he thought about Jani. He stopped for a moment then said, "It's not environmental. Stick with the Clozaril." At the time, the fellow resident working under Dr. Hyde showed us the latest research about Clozaril actually being able to repair part of the brain.

Now, Jani is getting better, Bodhi is getting worse, and I am beyond frustrated. Sure, Bodhi has autistic traits, but so does Jani and he's getting all the services for autism so why would it hurt to try Clozaril and see if it helps him? I decide to catch Dr. Hyde on his morning rounds to talk to him.

There he is! He walks past me sitting in the vestibule. He's like a God to me. I can't help it. He saved my daughter's life and now my son's life is on the line. "He's paranoid schizophrenic," I burst out, stopping Dr. Hyde in his tracks. He's holding his key card up to the magnetic strip that opens the electronic door.

I realize how crazy I must sound as he turns to face me. I recant my statement before he can respond. "Fine, he's autistic. When can we try Clozaril? Or at least Thorazine?" I am begging again. Thorazine is only given to him as a PRN. PRN is short for "pro re nata," which means when necessary. It's not used every day.

He looks back at me, about to confide something, but stops short. I sense that he knows more than he can tell me. When Bodhi was just shy of two, we shared an elevator ride down to the lobby. He couldn't help but look down at Bodhi in his stroller and study him for a moment, then look back up at me, his foreboding eyes telling me what I didn't want to know. At the time Bodhi was unmedicated. By the next time I saw him alone, Bodhi was on Risperdal and Dr. Hyde said, "He looks better now."

Here I am, some years later, waiting for his answer. "I can do Thorazine," is all he says as he disappears through the double doors.

*   *   *

Bodhi is discharged from the hospital on Jani's minimum day (early dismissal), so we all go to pick him up. This time he'll go straight from the hospital to his first appointment at UCLA's new on-site autism clinic.

I fill out Bodhi's discharge paperwork on the child psych unit while Michael and Jani wait for us at the clinic. Danielle, our social worker, asks the usual questions. "Do you have a gun in the home?"

"Nope."

"Do you keep the medicine out of reach?"

"Yep."

"And you'll make sure that he never leaves your sight?"

I find this last question hard to answer. "I have tons of people watching him all the time, but if you feel that he's not ready to be discharged then let me know."

"No, no," she half-laughs. "We're talking about parents who leave their kids alone and go shopping. Stuff like that."

"Oh God. No! I don't think Bodhi would be alive when I got back."

She nods. "Exactly."

We walk Bodhi over to the clinic with no pretense of politeness. In 2009, Danielle worked under Georgia, the Chief Social Worker. She confided that thirty years ago Jani would have been in the back ward of Camarillo State Hospital along with the other kids (twelve and under) diagnosed with schizophrenia. She'd also noticed Bodhi, running up and down the hallway, his head turned up like he was flying alongside a bird. "Watch him," Georgia said.

"Why?" I asked her, "What do you think?"

"He's looking up," she turns to me and we both stand, watching Bodhi. He isn't the least bit out of place in the psych ward. Even I can make the distinction between the kids here as visitors and those who are pa-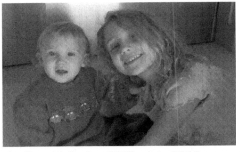

Bodhi with Jani at UCLA in 2009.

tients. Bodhi was always a patient. It just took four years for him to be admitted.

"All right, we're here," Danielle signs off, relieved at the sight of Michael and Jani ready to take over. I know we're not the easiest parents she's had to deal with but at least she's grown up with us.

We say our good-byes and walk into the kid-friendly room. We know we're in trouble when the first words out of Bodhi's mouth are "I want to go to Barnes & Noble!" but at least we made it safely to the autism clinic and we're on UCLA grounds.

"We can go to Barnes & Noble after your appointment." Michael is trying to calm him.

"Did you tell them we're here?" My eyes track the receptionist, nearly invisible under an elongated desk and other office equipment.

"Yes, but we have to wait a bit," he tells me, his eyes fixed on our son. "Bodhi, do you want to play with some toys? There are books and cars here…"

"I want to go to Target!" His voice speeds up. "Toys R Us…!"

Uh-oh, the flight of ideas. This is also associated with schizophrenia. "We will, Bodhi, we just have to go to your appointment here."

Bodhi crashes to the floor, his head arching back like an acrobat on meth. Jani moves aside, giving us the space we need. She's been through this so many times now. All she ever says is "he's schizophrenic."

Michael and I rush him over to the couch, automatically assuming our positions. The ever-present post-traumatic stress disorder (PTSD) comes over me and I yell to the receptionist, "We need the doctor NOW!"

"I paged him," she replies.

"Just hold him," Michael grits his teeth. Neither of us is nice at this point. We're soldiers on the battlefield, only responding to direct commands. I've got Bodhi's legs because that is my strength. Michael has the harder job, holding our son's head and arms, and he's already getting tired. Bodhi's mouth escapes Michael's grip, moving to the soft tissue between his own right thumb and forefinger. I take one hand off a leg, grabbing for his thumb, but I don't make it in time. Blood spurts out from the crevice.

"They said he was good to go." I panick. "WE NEED A DOCTOR!" Now I'm screaming, determined to get those damn doctors out of their foxholes.

Dr. Beta appears, his demeanor calm. He was once a fellow resident overseeing Jani's case. "He needs to go back," Michael says. "He's not ready to come home."

"We're going to help him here," Dr. Beta assures us. Michael and I are relieved when we see a familiar face, but he's just observing Bodhi, shocked and fascinated at the same time.

"I need medicine!" Bodhi cries out, clear as a bell. No speech delay.

"He needs medicine," I repeat Bodhi's own words back to Dr. Beta who appears to have not heard him.

"We're not pill-pushers here." He sits down on the couch a few inches away.

I laugh-cry. "You see what is going on here. Help him!" Another male doctor casually walks out to see what the fuss is about. Jani's bored so she's firing a million questions, then leads the doctor over to a small table where they look like a father and daughter talking about her day at school. Jani has become my hope and inspiration, but I'm shocked back to reality when I turn back to Bodhi, seeing more blue and purple bite marks popping up all over his arms, legs, and torso.

We've been going at it for a half-hour when this woman, a preppy flashback from the 80s, comes out with a heavy blanket. She speaks soothingly because of course, this is the whole problem: We're not talking quietly right now. She tries putting a blanket over him, but he kicks at her and she backs away. I think she's afraid. Why is she even working here? Isn't she used to this? This *is* the "autism clinic" after all.

As we soldier on, I know Bodhi's heart rate is rising, but the doctors always tell us not to worry because in children it's like they're running a marathon. *But how long can this marathon go on?* Bodhi grunts. "He needs to go to the bathroom," Michael looks up at me. "But there's no way I can take him alone. We have to call the paramedics!"

My mind flashes back to the news stories about how autistic

kids are tasered to get them under control. If Bodhi were in school and the teacher didn't know what to do, he would likely be one of those kids. Thank God we're here.

Dr. Beta's realizing that this is more serious than he thought. "I know. I called them." But moments later it's not the paramedics who arrive, it's UCLA Security followed by a policeman. Michael explains everything to the security guard who takes hold of Bodhi's head while Michael reconfigures himself to keep Bodhi's arms in place. I've still got his legs. The four of us, including Bodhi, are sweating profusely trying to keep him safe from himself. Even after all this time, he still hasn't received any medication.

"I need to take him to the bathroom," Michael looks up at the security guard. "That's part of his stress right now." So he and the security guard grab hold of Bodhi and slug him along, only to come back two minutes later. Michael frowns in disappointment. "We couldn't get him. He nearly cracked his skull on the urinal."

It's been over an hour and the paramedics haven't arrived. Meanwhile, parents of fearful autistic kids are being ushered out by security. The clinic is evacuated with guards remaining at the entrance to keep looky-loos away. "Didn't you call the paramedics?" I question Dr. Beta.

"Yes." He looks genuinely perplexed.

The policeman holds his walkie-talkie, calling the paramedics again as Bodhi rages, still going without the medication that he, himself, requested. We find out later that the paramedics were under the impression that this wasn't an emergency. And this is *another* big problem with the mental health care system. Because the mental health care parity laws are not given the same urgency, they don't get the same attention.

By the time the paramedics arrive, Michael decides he doesn't want Bodhi in restraints and holds him even after Bodhi's teeth dig deep into his skin leaving red dots circling welts. Jani and I meet Michael and Bodhi back at the ER where Dr. Beta encourages Michael to get a Tetanus shot. "I'm just so tired of going through this again," I tell Dr. Beta.

"It's not the same thing," he says. "You're going to have different challenges this time." And maybe he's right, but I'm not sure I want him to be. Jani's doing fine right now. Instead of looking at the same problem, knowing I will have the same outcome in five years, I may be looking at another problem with a different outcome. And will this outcome be better or worse?

CHAPTER 19

I BITE MYSELF

September 2013

Do I really want to do this? I'm tossing and turning, trying to get comfortable again, but can't fall back to sleep. I'm too restless. Bodhi was given another 300 milligrams of lithium before his last discharge, bringing him to a therapeutic level of 600 milligrams daily. He did great for a few weeks but it is late September and he is slipping again.

I walk into the living room and see Bodhi asleep on his twin bed, so I retreat back into what has become my bedroom. I know in my heart what I have to do but there's no way Michael is going to come with me and I don't want to put Jani through this again either. She'll understand why I'm not here when she wakes up.

I contemplate my next moves as I shower, then put on my most comfortable pajamas and slippers. I'm in for a hellishly long day but I have a plan this time. We waited at the ER all day yesterday only to be sent home last night because there were no beds available for Bodhi. His suitcase is still in the trunk of the car.

My mom called while I was driving home. I told her that his

heart rate went up to 170 but they didn't seem to think it was that serious. "Susan, you have to take him back!" My cellphone screams at me from the passenger seat. The panic in my mom's voice would make anyone think that she was in the back of the ER last night.

"I'm too tired," I yawn. "He's sleeping peacefully now. I can't go through this anymore. We told the doctors his heart rate went to 170, but they said it's like he's running a marathon."

"You HAVE to! His heart rate is too high. He could go into cardiac arrest!" *Cardiac arrest?!* "I don't like this, Susan." The shrillness in her voice is scaring me. "At least see a cardiologist."

A cardiologist?! Oh my God, what is this coming to? "Okay. I will take him tomorrow," I agree, ending the call and praying through my tears for God to guide me. His answer immediately strikes me like a lightning bolt, which is why, at 5 am, I'm back in the ER with Bodhi. He slept most of the way here but now he's awake, ramping up, fists banging together as he spins in small circles.

"Can I help you?" The triage nurse asks.

"Yes." I inhale a deep breath then exhale it before the race begins. "I need to see a cardiologist for my son. Yesterday, he was here waiting for a bed on the child psych unit. There wasn't one available, but that's not why I'm here," I lie easily because I have no choice. "His heart rate went up to 170 and my parents think he needs to see a cardiologist."

"Okay," she nods and I give her his name. Unlike Jani, whose name is one of her external triggers, Bodhi actually likes his name. But there's one word that sets him off every time so I know I won't have to wait long before the marathon begins.

"Come here, Bodhi," I brace myself.

The triage nurse unravels the blood pressure wrap.

On your mark....

She reaches over to Bodhi's bicep.

Get set....

"Can I take your 'vitals'?"

GO!

"AAAHHH!" He screams, arching his body back like a puppet dangling from the strings of a mad puppeteer.

"Does he need restraints?" The nurse comes alive.

"Yes," I say, keeping the pace as the ER doors fly open, my adrenalin at an all-time high, with two nurses now running alongside me, but this is just the warm-up. I need to reserve stamina to endure the cross-country portion of this run. I hop onto the gurney, keeping a strong hold on Bodhi while a middle-aged Hispanic male nurse squats to my left side and a twenty-something female nurse bring in soft nylon restraints, quickly wrapping them around all four sides of the bed's metal rods.

Bodhi and I share a moment of relief as he allows the intravenous needle to penetrate his vein. The medicine travels through his small body, giving him a momentary breather, before forcing his arm to tighten. Then...it's back!

His anguishing scream penetrates throughout both our bodies. I struggle to keep his jaw in place so he can't draw more of his own blood by biting down on his lower lip, but I lose my grip and Bodhi's teeth are now outlined in red. "I bite myself!" He cries, looking down at the crevice between his thumb and forefinger, the self-inflicted wound he gave himself in the autism clinic reopened, fresh blood squirting out.

"You're going to be okay," Bodhi," I say, without thinking. I can't think. If I do, I'll fall apart. So I speak softly and breathe hard. "I promise. You just need the right medication. Jani went through this too." I am talking to him but the words are to reassure me.

I lose hold and his mouth escapes me. Another bite mark indents the top of his shoulder, turning it purple. I feel like leaning into the male nurse beside me, resting for a moment but we're in the middle of a relay, all three of us. We take turns passing around the white washcloth, soaked in blood. Instead, "Do you have children?" I ask him, trying to keep myself from shaking.

"Yeah," he says, a tear forming in the corner of his eye. He's sweating but manages to keep Bodhi's arms in place while the female nurse keeps hold of his little legs. The restraints are not enough.

"Do you have children?" I ask her too.

She looks up, unable to hide her tears because her hands aren't free to wipe them off her face. "I have a five-year-old daughter." These two nurses are feeling what I am in this moment: animalistic fear. My eyes shift over to the heart monitor. Bodhi's heart rate is 180 and climbing!

I lift my head from the frenzy to catch my breath and my mind drifts off for a second. Am I really here? Sitting behind the baby boy I gave birth to over five years ago? I carried him around, protected him from everything, kept him safe in my arms.

I'm jolted back as searing pain shoots through me. Oh my God, my index finger is caught in his mouth! I can't get it out! I jiggle it as hard as I can while the male nurse helps free it from Bodhi's clenched teeth. It's finally free, with blood surfacing around the numb edges of my fingernail. I'm furious, but not with Bodhi. These worthless doctors are nowhere to be found, even though I see them at the nurses' station just outside our door.

His heart monitor machine is beeping so I look over at it: 202! My son's heart rate is now 202! I jam my right hand down on the intercom. They're not coming fast enough! I do it again, and again. I won't stop. "My son's going into CARDIAC ARREST!" I am yelling, again. "I need a DOCTOR!!!"

A pack of scrubs shows up, one coming to my side. "You need to calm down, Ma'am." The others look him over as a woman dressed in regular clothes clicks toward me, her heels an unmistakable marker: She is another social worker. Unbelievably, except that it isn't, she asks if I would like coffee or tea. Useless.

"NO! I need a DOCTOR!!"

"The doctor's right here," she nods to the side of her. My eyes narrow in on a petite woman that may as well be dressed in a Catholic school girls' uniform and burst out. "She's the doctor?!"

"I just gave him another 12.5 milligrams of Thorazine." She talks like a small child. I can barely hear her. *No wonder I didn't notice her before.*

"Twelve-point-five? That's nothing. He can go up to 100 milligrams and even that won't guarantee he'll calm down enough." Twenty-five milligrams can knock down an adult man for the night. I look at the IV in Bodhi's right arm. It is stained with new and old blood from when we first got here, but he doesn't complain. He's already learned that he has to go through this trauma before he can get some relief and become himself again. Until the next time.

I call Michael and tell him where we are. "I thought you would be there," he says, with a hint of sarcasm. He acts like I'm giving Bodhi a new toy that he was supposed to wait for until his birthday.

*   *   *

"You let them put him in restraints?!" Michael is so angry, as if it's somehow my fault. It's 1 pm and we're still in the same place we were since early this morning. He brought Jani and our friend Scarlet with him. We've known Scarlet for a while now. She's very meek but she, too, has schizophrenia and she lives close by. She reached out to us on Facebook after she saw our story on Oprah. She's been a godsend, helping us with Jani and Bodhi. Really, she's the best help we've ever had and she does it for her own therapy.

"I didn't know what else to do. You don't want to come with me anymore. Do you know his heart rate went up to 202?!"

"Well, are they going to admit him?" Michael asks. He's becoming less helpful with each hospitalization.

"Yes, they're going to admit him."

Chapter 20

Changing the Guard

Fall 2013

I love sleeping and, once again, I feel guilty about getting a good night's sleep while Bodhi's inpatient, but this is my reality. The same reality I lived—we lived—when Jani was in the hospital. It wasn't until Jani started Clozaril that her sleeping habits became what they are today, nearly twelve hours a night. During this time, while they're in-patient, I'm also able to think more clearly.

"We need to change behaviorists," I tell Michael. "The ones we have right now aren't working for Jani. I need her to be able to shower in the morning so I can focus on getting Bodhi ready for school. It's nearly impossible to manage both kids alone in the morning."

"I'm up all night grading." His silent resentment screams at me, as though I'm accusing him of something. Nothing is ever easy between us anymore.

"I know. This is why we need a new team who can work around us. We shouldn't have to work around their schedules. I just need someone, obviously female, to help Jani take her showers."

"Yvette said she can do that."

"But her schedule's inconsistent. She's trying to teach Jani to take a shower at all different times of the day."

"That's because she's going to college."

"I know that. The problem is that we shouldn't be working around her schedule. She should be working around OURS!"

"Why are you always yelling at me?!"

"Because I feel like I have to fight *you* on top of everyone else!"

"You expect too much from people."

"You're right. I do." I take a moment to reflect on this deep thought coming from my husband who is being an asshole. "I guess I never thought about it that way."

"Good. I'm glad you see that."

I nod. "We just need someone to help get Jani into a morning routine before school."

"Fine. But what about Bodhi? He'll have to get used to all new people. They usually don't change all at once."

"This is going to happen before he gets out of the hospital, and the new team agreed to meet him *in* the hospital."

"Okay, whatever."

*   *   *

"I don't want them watching me!" Jani is shouting at one of the stricter adaptive therapists on the new team. They go under a different title because of Jani's age but really, it's all the same thing.

"Then you need to take a shower by yourself." I stand beside her shower warden. "Do you want people *always* watching you?"

"No," she answers.

"This is why you need to do it yourself."

Hygiene is one of the most serious problems for people with schizophrenia because they're often so disconnected from their bodies. When Jani was eight months old, we were at the park and she was climbing up this metal structure. I rested my arm on it then instantly jerked it away. It was hot! Very hot! I'd told my mom and she said that it wasn't normal. It didn't go any further than that but now I look back and realize the significance.

*   *   *

Bodhi always comes home from the hospital filled with anxiety. This is the normal adjustment period. We pick him up late in the afternoon so we have less of the day to get through. We prepare dinner but he's refusing to take his meds.

Thank God for the knock at our door. It's Devon, the new team supervisor, with Alysha and Daria, the shadows she is training to take over. Daria has a very sophisticated beauty about her and seems especially smart with her clipboard in hand. It is clear she has more experience in the field than Alysha. Then, there's Devon, she's the supervisor. "So, how's he doing?" Devon's energy is strong, having trained as a ballerina. She looks and acts the part.

"He won't take his medicine."

She plants a smile on her face, guiding her team toward the kitchen table. "Okay, here's what we're going to do…" she gathers her long hair into a ponytail even a pony would envy. Bodhi is eating his chicken nuggets and French fries. "First, we're going to make a list of everything he likes," she directs her smile to me and Bodhi, while bringing out a stream of papers from her notebook. "Then we can find out which things he wants in the moment, whether it be the iPad, cars, snacks…whatever. These are what we'll use later to barter with him. And if we have to," she takes a deep breath. "We'll bring it down to even smaller steps."

She turns her attention to Bodhi. "Bodhi, do you remember me from the hospital?" Bodhi doesn't say anything but looks in her direction. "Do you know my name?"

"Devon."

"Yes, very good." She smiles at us. "He's got a great memory."

"He knows everything," I tell her. "He only talks when he really wants to."

"Well, that's what we will work on." Her manner reassures me.

135

Bodhi gets up from his seat and walks over to the pantry. He brings out packaged fruit snacks and comes to me. "Open these."

I'm about to open them when Devon puts her hand up to stop me. "You need to take your medicine first," she tells Bodhi. A rush of excitement comes over me as I follow her order. I hand her the fruit snacks and prepare a new cup of juice with his medicine. Jani just swallows pills so this was never an issue, but Bodhi will only take them in his juice and lately, he's been refusing that. He takes the cup from me, drinks a little, then lets it drool down the sides of his chin.

I look to Devon to take charge. She opens the packet of fruit snacks and shows Bodhi what he'll get if he takes his medicine. "We'll use one fruit snack in exchange for one sip," she says. The other girls watch closely as Devon twirls her fingers around the straw inside the plastic cup. She is completely focused on Bodhi and the box of fruit snacks in front of him. "Just one sip...and you can have one fruit snack."

Bodhi takes a sip, but the red juice slides down his chin again. We all sigh, disappointed, as he cries. "Let's try this again," she says, while Daria reaches for a napkin to wipe his chin. "Which *color* fruit snack do you want?"

He studies them. "Red."

"Okay. Just swallow one sip of your medicine and you can have the red one." The cup is offered and he takes another sip. More drool and another wipe of his chin. "Bodhi, let's try a smaller sip."

He takes a smaller sip and it goes down. Devon is satisfied and gives him the red fruit snack. "Have you ever thought of hiding it in his food?" Daria asks.

"Yes, if I have to, but I'd rather he know what medicine he's taking because if it turns out that he's actually paranoid schizophrenic then the last thing I want to do is add to his paranoia." They nod while their eyes stay fixated on the exchange between Devon and Bodhi. After about 45 minutes of trading one fruit snack for one sip, the cup is empty.

*   *   *

Another change I make is with Bodhi's respite care. Correll is fantastic and accompanies me out with Bodhi but she can no longer control him alone. He may be small, but he's strong and even stronger when his symptoms flare. The whole purpose of respite is for Michael and me to get a break, even go out, but this has become impossible because Bodhi requires a strong male who can gently restrain him if need be.

I call Bill, our vendor at the regional center that contracts their services. Correll warns me that he's very dramatic. "I have the perfect guy for you! He's tall and strong with a good head on his shoulders. He's a basketball player. You're going to love him!" Obviously, Bill has fallen for this new guy but I am a little hesitant. This is not a job for the weak and our next step is re-acclimating Bodhi back into a school routine.

Devon and her team are here bright and early, ready to begin their session with Bodhi. Michael has to take Jani to school because I can't leave the apartment without triggering Bodhi into a major meltdown. Jani has always been Daddy's girl, but Bodhi is definitely Momma's boy.

There's a knock at the door. I ask Devon if it's another team member, but she says everyone's here. At this point in our lives, the apartment manager likens our place to that of drug traffickers because so many people are always coming and going.

"Who is it?"

"Zach. I'm here for respite."

"Oh yeah. That's right!" I turn to Devon and her team, putting everyone at ease. "He's our new respite for Bodhi," I say, opening the door as he bends down to shake my hand. He's so tall and it's very early in the morning but I feel rejuvenated at the sight of this Adonis standing before me.

I look over at the other girls and I'm clearly not alone in my assessment, or Bill's for that matter. He's *gorgeous*! For the first time in years, I'm distracted. I think somewhere along the line I forgot what it felt like to be a woman, to have this feeling come over me.

"Nice to meet you." I feel like a schoolgirl. *I'm almost 44. How is this possible?*

"I'm here for Bodhi." I invite him in, forgetting for a moment where Bodhi went. Thankfully, I have help from the girls because my mind just took an unexpected trip out of Holland, to another country entirely. We all become quick friends and Bodhi immediately bonds to Zach.

"So, you're just respite?" Devon asks, like he should be way higher on the totem pole. Behaviorists are paid twice what respite is.

"Yeah. I'm a basketball player," he says, solemnly. "I was going for the NBA until I was injured during a game. When I lost my scholarship at Santa Barbara, I just came back home." He sounds so disheartened that we all feel bad for him.

"Well, we're glad to have you here," I say, grateful to see this gentle giant standing before me.

CHAPTER 21

NEW AT THIS

November 2013

We all meet at Old Orchard's school playground, the same school where Jani is a 5th grader. Michael and I discuss the logistics and decide he will drop Jani off in the valet while I follow with Bodhi, Daria, and Zach. I make sure to keep my distance, letting Daria and Zach take over on the playground. To the average eye, Bodhi looks like any other kindergartner, playing on the jungle gym and needing some assistance with the swings. The hope is that eventually he'll feel comfortable enough for me to leave entirely.

When the bell rings, I accompany the new team to Bodhi's classroom where he settles in playing alongside another boy and girl. They share building blocks and everything is going along smoothly, until they're told to take their seats. I remain where I am, watching Daria and Zach guide Bodhi to his desk. He's a little fidgety, but maybe, just maybe, he'll make it with two people shadowing him.

Daria and Zach are on either side of him, enticing him with crayons to stay seated, as the final bell rings. Ms. Kristen tells the class to be seated and within seconds Bodhi arches back, screaming.

SHIT!

"Maybe it's better if I go into the office?" My teammates nod and I walk into the office just in time to see Michael coming in after dropping Jani off in the valet. We sit and watch the clock. Every minute that ticks by we look at each other, silently praying to get to that next minute.

"AAAHHH…." The familiar scream.

"He's not gonna make it." Michael's defeated tone infuriates me.

"What do you mean? Don't you remember going through this with Jani?"

"Not like this."

"Yes, it was different in some ways, but he's also a boy. He's not as verbal as she was."

"He's going to have to go to a special program." I know what Michael's thinking. He wants Bodhi to go to "The Help Group" in Sherman Oaks. Not that they're bad. I've actually heard they're very good, but the Newhall School District is where he's familiar. Our behaviorists wouldn't be able to go with him and he would be more than a half hour away. *What if something happened there?*

"*No!* I want him close to us. I don't trust other programs where we can't be near him."

"You don't trust anyone," Michael turns on me.

"You're right. I don't because he's not their son. He's MY son!"

"He's my son too. And I can't do this anymore!"

"Fine. Then don't. I will." I get up, meeting Daria and Zach coming into the office.

"He's having a hard time but we're getting through it." Zach's words comfort me. *Oh, how I want to fall into his strong arms.* I'm so lucky to have him here at this time, when Michael is falling apart. He and Daria have other cases and need to leave. I excuse Daria, then tell Michael. "Zach is riding home with Bodhi and me."

Michael's shoulders slump. "I need a moment anyway," he says before he walks across the street to our other car. Maybe he noticed something in the way I talk about Zach or look at him. It's not like he is never interested in other women.

"It's okay. I'll meet you at home. Zach, can you sit in the back with Bodhi?"

"Sure," he says, helping Bodhi into the back seat. I drive extra carefully because I can't help looking back at them to make sure Bodhi is okay. Zach is cuddling him while I tremble like a teenager. I don't know what to say to make conversation so I turn on the radio. "What are you going to do now?" he asks.

I come back out of my fantasy world and talk to Zach's soulful light brown eyes through the rearview mirror. They look so engaging, loving, and concerned. "We have another behaviorist coming over, but if he's not better by tomorrow morning, I'll have to take him back to the hospital. Can you come with me?"

"I think so. I just have to text Bill and make sure I'm available." He starts texting, and I start praying. "I can do it." I breathe a sigh of relief.

Thank you, God.

*   *   *

As expected, Bodhi's goes all night and Michael refuses to get up, so I spend the very early part of the morning packing Bodhi's suitcase with comfy clothes, cars, and small plastic train sets. When Daria arrives at six, Michael's still sleeping so I tell her my plan. We need to get Jani to school without upsetting her schedule. She's doing well and the last thing I need is for her to start decompensating. I know that me not being here is going to trigger Bodhi, but I have to make a choice right now and Jani has to come first in this moment. Besides, one of Bodhi's goals is to be able to separate from me. Right now, I'm trapped inside my own home.

By the time I get back, Michael is furious. "Why did you leave?! Bodhi's screaming and biting himself. We've been in restraint for half an hour. *I* could have taken Jani to school!"

"You were sleeping," I reply, calmly, as I see Daria holding Bodhi's legs. "Let me get the liquid Benadryl." I race over to the cupboards then back over to them. "Keep his mouth open long enough to pour some in."

"When he bites down," Daria instructs me, "rub your finger sideways between his nose and upper lip." She demonstrates. "It's an automatic reflex action that will force his jaw to open." I wish I'd known that before.

There's a knock at the door. "Come in!" I am relieved at the sight of Zach charging into the game, playing defense against Bodhi battling...Bodhi. Michael is still holding onto Bodhi's head and I've got his feet, while Zach grabs his arms,

"You got 'em?" Daria asks Zach, like she's handing over weights at the gym.

"Yeah," he says, relieving Daria to write her session notes.

"Tell Devon that I'm taking him back to UCLA today."

"Okay," she swallows hard. No questions asked. I turn to Michael. "All I need you to do is pick up Jani."

"That's fine." Michael's nearly out of breath, handing Bodhi over to Zach. "I need a moment." He goes for his cigarettes above the refrigerator. Apparently, he was about to have one before My Bodhi Tree was uprooted.

"Can you hold him for a moment?" I ask Zach as Michael takes his cigarette onto the balcony. I just love how Zach can keep Bodhi safe in his arms.

It's going to be a long day so I go into the bedroom and change into more comfortable clothes. I'm in the middle of removing my bra when Zach comes in to ask me something. He stops short and my mind takes flight again. I'm tired of being strong. I want someone else to be strong and hold me together, even just for a little while. But instead, Zach just looks at me as I continue getting dressed. I have no idea what question he asked or even what I answered.

*　　*　　*

This ride to UCLA is different. My eyes wander up to the rearview mirror where I see Zach in the back seat. It is a relief to have Bodhi safe in his arms. It's not like I don't get what Michael is feeling. I do, but when he's weak, I have no choice but to be the stronger one. I just want strong, loving arms around me for once.

Bodhi has been doing well during the ride, giving us a reprieve from his thrashing. I'm easily able to park in the valet lot outside the emergency room. Bodhi knows everything. Even he feels relieved to be back at UCLA. I hand my keys to the valet in exchange for a ticket, then assume my new role as Zach's coach as we move through the automatic doors and approach the triage nurse.

"Be prepared for anything," I whisper in his ear as he holds Bodhi in his arms. This is a different nurse from the one I had a couple months back so I just relax and let it all happen.

"Can I take your vitals?" she asks.

"AAAHHH!" Bodhi springs backward, but Zach is prepared. I'm so glad he was an athlete. I'm sorry he got injured, ruining his chances for the NBA, but this game is a matter of life and death and hopefully, it will carry more meaning for him in the long run.

The ER door swings open and Bodhi is back in attack mode. Zach holds onto him like a basketball, only this basketball is biting at his arms. I'm blocking his side, trying to keep Bodhi's head in one place so he can't chomp down. Zach looks over at the nursing station. "Why aren't they helping us?" His moist eyes bare his soul and it dawns on me that I'm so desensitized that I didn't even notice.

"They never do," I tell him. "That's why I wanted you here with me." Zach's tearing up and I cry with him. He can't physically stop Bodhi from chomping down on his skin while we're being led to the back ward, a place I've spent so many hours before.

We get Bodhi down on the examining table and he's still flailing around with all his might. "We need restraints!" I call out to whoever's in earshot. Both Zach and I are now committed to keeping Bodhi from doing more damage to his body and Zach's. It's a workout, and we are rolling around on top of the examining table.

"Can you scratch my shoulder," Zach asks, tears streaming

down his cheeks. He's so sensitive, warm, and loving. Finally, a nurse comes in with restraints and I tell her he needs medication.

The actual nurse robot-eyes the situation. "I have to check with the doctor." She comes back. "It says he can't have Thorazine."

"I know, but we need *something*." I am crying, struggling to keep Bodhi steady in Zach's arms. The last time he went inpatient, he was withdrawing from Risperdal and two nurses believed Thorazine was making him worse. I know it was the withdrawal from Risperdal, but they didn't believe me.

The nurse whisks herself away like this is just part of her day, which I suppose it is. "I can't believe no one is here to help us." Zach is in a state of shock, the same shock I'd gone through the first time with Jani. Now, I'm familiar with "the game," but at 21, Zach is still new to this.

CHAPTER 22

PAPER TRAIL

November 2012

"You can't keep taking him to the hospital," Dr. Howe warns us. We're in her office a week before Thanksgiving. Not even a month has passed since Bodhi's been outpatient.

"Then he needs to be on the right medication," I argue.

She shakes her head. "He looks like he's doing fine to me."

"That's because the Seroquel works for a while then just stops working." I get tired of explaining the same thing, over and over.

"Susan's right," Michael backs me up this time. "He's fine now, but he can turn on a dime and then he's back in a self-harm state. We think it's because he's growing…."

"I don't think he's on the right medication." I know it makes Michael mad when I say that, but I don't care anymore.

"That's because he's schizophrenic," Jani adds, making Dr. Howe purse her lips.

"Would you stop saying that?!" Michael bares his teeth at me. "We don't know what he has yet."

"I didn't say it."

"Yeah, but you allow her to say it."

Uggghhh. "So, what do we do when he gets out of control again?" I look to Dr. Howe.

"Give him Benadryl, but only 12.5 milligrams per hour."

"That's not going to do anything," Michael says. Thank God we still agree on some things.

"You don't know what it's like!" I tell her, my voice, desperate. "In these moments he's practically killing himself!"

"Then here's what I want you to do," Dr. Howe advises. "Every time he's out of control, call the paramedics to start a paper trail."

*　　*　　*

I have no choice but to make the call. "Do you go through this with all your clients?" I ask Devon, perspiring, our clothes sticking to our skin from the effort it takes to keep Bodhi restrained. Her petite ballerina legs cover Bodhi's calves. She keeps his arms gently crossed over each other behind his back while I hold a blanket under his chin so when his jaw is free he'll bite the blanket, not himself.

"Yes...and...no," she breathes out, as though she is rehearsing for *The Nutcracker*.

"So, you've never had a case like this?" I press, just to make sure I'm not crazy.

"Most of them...will tire themselves out," she wriggles around with me, keeping Bodhi contained. "After an hour," she exhales, "they go to sleep." She closes her eyes, holding a tight smile. "They don't keep going like this."

"Dr. Howe says I should I should call the paramedics and start a paper trail. Do you think I should call them now? We're going on three hours."

"Yes," she says, her body twisted into a human straight-jacket.

*　　*　　*

When the paramedics arrive, they carefully muscle Bodhi into an orange papoose and I ride with him to Henry Mayo hospital where, after more hours of restraint in the same orange papoose, his heart

146

rate is rising. Alone now, I solemnly sit with him, emotionally and physically drained.

"Do you need anything?" An older, balding male nurse comes in to check on us.

"No," I shake my head, too worn out to feel anything. Then I stop him. "Have you ever seen a case like this?" When I put myself in "interview-mode," I can disconnect from the situation and gain the necessary strength to move forward.

"Not this severe."

I can't believe it. I thought Jani was supposed to be the most severe case? What the hell is happening here?! "You know," I feel the tension in my voice rising, "what you're doing here is torture!" He follows my eyes over to Bodhi, a little boy strapped to a gurney, screaming, clenching his fists together like he's been in a war and part of his body needs to be amputated.

"You're right."

"I want the doctor to try Haldol," I instruct him, knowing that both Dr. Howe and Dr. Hyde are never going to approve it, especially after the false report that Thorazine was causing his agitation. Bodhi is suffering because two nurses decided I was a Crazy Mom. If they had considered the Risperdal withdrawal like I told them, he might have been heading toward the right medication.

So, instead, I request a medication that has never been tried on Bodhi and pray for the best. Haldol sent Jani into dystonia years ago, but that was because Dr. Howe never told us to give it to her with Benadryl or Cogentin. Unfortunately, we never got to that point, because she was immediately taken off Haldol and put on Zyprexa. That worked for a while before she tried jumping out of her bedroom window.

The ER doctor calls Howe and Hyde, but neither one returns the call, leaving it up to him. "I'd like to try Phenergan first and if that doesn't work, we'll try Haldol." At least he's trying something. Bodhi's IV is slowly injected with this cough medicine. As I watch it seep into his veins, his arms tense up, his fists clenching so hard that they're turning purple and his teeth are chattering.

"It's not working!" I run up to the doctor sitting at the nursing station. "Please come and see him!" He follows me back to Bodhi's room, looks at the monitor and tells the nurse that they're going to try the Haldol with Benadryl.

The doctor, nurse, and I stand, eyes glued to the monitor, as Bodhi's body slowly unwinds. His balled fists release themselves and his fingers are stretch out. We wait with bated breath as Bodhi's heart rate begins to drop from dangerously high levels.

I fall over, crying in relief, as the doctor and nurse exchange hopeful glances. We all took a chance and it worked. Bodhi is tired, but he's back.

After six hours wrapped in a papoose, strapped to a hospital bed, they begin taking out the intravenous needle and unraveling the restraints, setting him free from the modern-day straight jacket he's worn since Devon and I made the call.

*   *   *

I page Dr. Howe as Correll and I sit on the benches watching Bodhi wriggle around like a breaching whale at Academy Swim. He's usually so good in the water! He's a natural swimmer but it's been a few minutes and today is not looking good. "The medicine is not working again and I already gave him the full dose." I turn to Correll and she nods, sympathetically, as Dr. Howe returns my page.

"Well, if you gave him the full dosage, then you just blew your whole wad!" She is screaming at me. Then, dial tone.

"She hung up on me?" My mouth drops open. Correll tightens her lips as we watch Bodhi taking off his trunks in the water. Oh God, now he's swimming naked. "I can't give him any more. He's already had his prescribed dose. I don't know what to do?" We barely make it home with Correll in the back seat, doing her best to block Bodhi's moves during the drive. I call Michael, preparing him for the inevitable restraint. It's only Saturday. How do we get through Sunday?

"We...can't...call the paramedics again," Michael stresses, doing his best to carry Bodhi from the car into our apartment. The three of us carry him onto his bed in the living room. Correll uses her own body, as though she's in the middle of doing push-ups over Bodhi.

"We have to." I am making the call. "Besides, Dr. Howe wants us to start a paper trail." But when the paramedics arrive, they're not alone. Two police officers accompany them, and they don't look happy. They start questioning us on why we've called them to our home two days in a row. We tell them what happened, and thank God that we have Correll to back it up because I'm beginning to feel uneasy about this whole "paper trail" we're starting.

In late afternoon, we get word at Henry Mayo that there are no beds available at UCLA. *There's a shocker.* I'm curious, so I ask, "Is there another hospital that *does* have a bed?" And of course, the answer is yes: BHC Alhambra has a bed. I cry my story to a young nurse who is empathetic because her parents went through similar trials with her younger brother who has Down's syndrome.

"Hold on," she tells me, then disappears for a while. When she comes back, she reassures me that she's doing her best to help.

About two hours later, Dr. Jack comes in. He's a handsome man who appears to be in his mid-30s and at the top of his game. He's read Bodhi's file and understands the need for him to go back to UCLA. "Give me a few minutes," he calms me with a smile. "I teach the fellows at UCLA and I know one of the nurses there. I might be able to work something out." Oh my God. This is unheard of, especially on a Saturday.

"Okay," I say, leaving it up to fate, thinking about Chanel and Chelsee. Both are guardian angels on the unit. They even caught me filming one of Bodhi's episodes, but because Michael and I were giving them a reprieve at the time, they just looked at each other, dark circles around their eyes, and walked away. They love Bodhi. Most of the nurses there do but the problem is me, not the kids. I'm too "assertive," or probably downright bitchy, so a lot of the nurses don't like me and may deny this request so they don't have to deal with me.

I watch as Dr. Jack talks to the Henry Mayo nurse then moves on to another patient. The nurse picks up the phone, so I slip out of the room, listening in on the conversation. "Which nurse are you talking to?"

"I'm not sure," she tells me. "I'm on hold."

I go back to Bodhi's room and stare at the walls. I've always hated hospitals. Michael says he could live in one. Jani likes them too, and it's starting to look like Bodhi is also comfortable around all the equipment, especially when he's in a manic state. So, I guess it's just me. I don't want to live in a hospital, mental or otherwise. I'm too claustrophobic.

*   *   *

By evening, Dr. Jack returns. "I'm still waiting for a call back." Bodhi is sleeping between episodes, but just like at home, once he's awake, we're counting down the minutes before it will begin again. I press Dr. Jack for more information about Bodhi getting a bed.

"I'm 99 percent sure." I burst into tears, emotionally and physically drained. At least Michael is at home with Jani. I have no idea what I would do if I were a single mom. I'm so grateful to have him, to have help. "Thank you, God." The nurse comes back in and checks Bodhi's vitals. Fortunately, he is calm and doesn't mind them being taken.

"Which nurse were you talking to?"

"That was Chanel." My eyes close and tears stream down my cheeks. It's amazing how when you just close your eyes, the world becomes more peaceful. My prayers were answered. "She's going to do some maneuvering around. We'll transport him from here by ambulance." I'm dizzy with glee. This time, I will NOT let them release him unless he is completely stable. I don't care how long it takes. Not after all we've gone through and all he's had to endure.

This is torture.

PART THREE

CHAPTER 23

GOODNIGHT, HONEY

January 8th, 2014

"Honey had a seizure." Michael stands before my bed and I sit up without thinking. If it's not one thing, it's another.

Bodhi just got out of the hospital after six weeks inpatient. He's on a higher dosage of Seroquel now and it appears to be working. At least he's sleeping better. I follow Michael into the hallway where we sit with Honey, her fifteen-year-old body trembling, her eyes rolling over. *This is it.*

"I'm going to take her to the vet," Michael wells up.

"I know." I let my tears flow. It's hard for me to cry these days because of all the meds I'm taking to keep myself together. They help me not cry so I can function every day. But when the pain is too overwhelming, I manage to release the tears. And I need this release. We've been preparing for this moment for a couple years now, but it doesn't make it any easier.

"What are we going to tell Jani?"

"We have to tell her the truth."

I hug Honey close and kiss her all over. "I love you, Honey." I know this is the last time I will ever hold her, but right now she's still breathing air and I'm happy to have this time with her.

* * *

Michael calls me from the vet's office and I get to tell her how much I've always loved her. "She hears you," Michael is crying over the phone. After he hangs up, I wallow in bed, waiting for his next call. The Call. I reminisce over our lives up until this point. How much we've been through. Honey was always by our side.

A few minutes later, his call comes in. "She's gone," he says, softly. We share a long cry over the phone, reliving years of memories. "She went peacefully. The doctor didn't need much morphine," He replays the night for me. "I even gave her a chance to go back before we got down to the car. I asked her if she wanted to go back upstairs, or to the vet," he hard-swallows. "She got into the car and laid down on the floor, just like when you brought her home that first night."

"She had a good life. I was happy when she made it to ten, then eleven, twelve, thirteen, fourteen, and fifteen. Remember, she had a problem with her liver when we first got her?"

"Yeah, I do." He sniffs. "They're going to cremate her and send us the ashes." Then, he takes another deep breath. "I called Scarlet. I'm going to pick her up so she can help with Jani."

"Yes, that's a great idea." Scarlet will help soften the blow for Jani and Bodhi.

* * *

I can't even lift my head off the pillow when Friday sneaks into my bedroom later that night. When Honey was thirteen, the vet told us she only had a couple more years to live. At the time, Jani and Michael were volunteering at the animal shelter. They first saw this beautiful Border Collie on a Friday. We introduced him to Honey and they liked each other immediately, making us wish we'd gotten another dog for her sooner. At least she had him as a companion and playmate for the last two years of her life.

I hear him curl up on the floor in the corner of the room like Honey used to, but when morning comes I open my eyes to find that it's not Friday, it's Scarlet. I forgot she was coming. "I thought you were Friday," I tell her, still shaking off the shock of losing Honey, and of finding her on the floor of my bedroom.

She gives a soft, sad laugh. "I didn't want to wake you." Scarlet and I have grown closer over the past year. She's like a sister to me. She says that caring for Jani is like therapy to keep her own schizophrenia under control. She helps me with Bodhi too. Her body is tinier than Devon's but she knows how to configure herself to do the proper restraint.

"Every morning when Jani gets up," I tell Scarlet, "she looks for Honey to make sure she's here. This time, she won't be."

"That's why *I'm* here, Sweetie," Scarlet gives me a sheepish smile. She stands up in the same clothes she slept in last night and we both go out into the living room. The apartment feels weird. Different. Less than.

"I'm going to take a shower now," I get my routine together. "Jani's adaptive therapist will be here soon and I have to prepare myself."

"Go ahead," Scarlet waves me on. Michael is a rolled-up ball on the floor, but he suffered the most last night. He did the hard work. I have to be strong now and give him time to sleep.

*　　　*　　　*

We're lucky because it's not just Jani's adaptive therapist who comes this morning. Her supervisor Annette comes too, giving us more people to protect Jani from what she could do in an impulsive state. I walk into Jani's room with her adaptive therapists behind me. I make sure she takes her morning meds before she takes a shower. Usually, I do it afterwards, but today I want them to take effect as soon as possible.

I'm relieved that Michael thought to bring Scarlet because she's able to keep Bodhi entertained while we focus on Jani. Bodhi loved

Honey too, but it's not the same. He never had the kind of bond with Honey that Jani had. I remember Honey guarding Jani in her infant car seat on the porch of our Burbank apartment. As Jani got older, she played vet to whatever pretend injury Honey had. She was incredibly patient with Jani, more so than a "normal" dog might be.

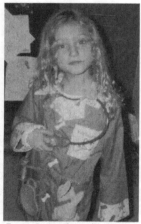

After we got Friday, we came to realize that Honey, too, has "special needs" and we just automatically accommodated them. Who knew she would be this much preparation for Jani and now Bodhi too? Friday is so neuro-typical, it is weird. He even wags his tail when we come home. Honey would bark and leap up on us, pounding us with her paws. We got used to it and were surprised when Friday didn't do this and just let people come in. Sure, he sniffs them and walks around them a bit but that's it.

Jani dressed up as a vet for Halloween 2007.

When Jani comes out of her room, she immediately sees Scarlet as the rest of us create a wide circle around her. "Hi-yee, Jani." Scarlet often lingers her words, especially when she's nervous, but she smiles sweetly at Jani, giving me time to think about how to answer the inevitable question coming my way.

"What are we going to do today, Mommy?"

"Well, Daddy had a long night, so Scarlet and I are going to take you and Bodhi to the Burbank Mall since it's close to Dr. Howe's office. Then we have to go to your appointments."

Jani looks around for Honey. She's been doing this for the past year. She begins in the kitchen then walks over to the bathroom. This is where Honey slept most of the time over the past year. "Where's Honey?"

"Honey passed away last night," I say, bluntly, knowing there's no other way to answer this. Jani's eyes drift off to the side, trying to process this. "Daddy took her to the vet and I was even able to talk to her over the phone. She died in Daddy's arms, just like in

Marley & Me." We'd all watched this movie a hundred times during Honey's last year. Even though we knew the ending, it never stopped us from crying.

Long seconds go by....

"Okay," she finally says. "We have to get another dog." This is Jani's answer to everything. Whenever one of her fish died Michael would go to the pet store with her to get a new one. The same with her turtles, if one passed on, we were back at the animal shelter, rescuing another one, but it's more complicated with a dog.

"Jani, this is why we have Friday."

"I know," she says, trying to work through this. We're all holding our breath, should she take off screaming, running out the door. "But...*eventually*," she stresses the word.

"Yes...eventually. But right now you have Friday and he needs lots of love because he misses Honey too."

"Aww, Friday," she drops to her knees and wraps her arms around his neck, nuzzling him close to her. We all breathe easier, her adaptive therapists impressed, as they've seen Jani at her worst. I close my eyes, grateful to God that this went as well as it did. Honey died peacefully, having given our family so much more than I could have ever expected the first night I saw her.

*   *   *

"I don't know how I could do this without you," I tell Scarlet. She is sitting in the backseat, holding Bodhi close to her. Driving with him is still tenuous. It's ironic how it used to be Jani and now it's reversed.

"Of coourrsse," she lingers. "I'm here for you. You're family."

Jani fiddles with the car radio looking for a song she can sing along to, but the first one triggers Bodhi. "I like that song," he says, following up with an angry, "I DON'T like that song!" *Uh-oh.* Bodhi does this a lot. He'll say something then recant the statement, like when he screams, "I feel better," then a second later comes, "I DON'T feel better!"

"Okay, Bodhi." I press the button to change the station. Both our cars are over a decade old and the CD players stopped working years ago. Bodhi likes most music so if I just change it up he'll usually be fine and, thankfully, Jani goes along with it.

When we get to the Burbank Mall, I pull into an open space near Barnes & Noble and IKEA. Jani leaps out of the car, ready to start her routine. "I want to go to McDonald's." She amazes me with how well she's handling the death of Honey. None of us has even had a moment to grieve.

"Okay." I look over at Scarlet, following Jani out of the car. "Bodhi, do you want to go to McDonald's?"

"No. Aaahhh!!!" He screams, falling to the ground.

SHIT! I just gave him his Seroquel and it is not working! He needs a stronger anti-psychotic, but I have to follow doctor's orders. "Okay," I say, thinking fast on my feet. "Scarlet, why don't you take Jani to McDonald's and I'll take Bodhi to Barnes & Noble." I bring Bodhi back up to a standing position, only to have him collapse beneath me again.

"Are you sure you can do this, Susan?" Scarlet stands, frozen in the middle of the parking lot, mirroring my helplessness.

"I want to go to McDonald's!" Jani uses routine to hold on to her own sanity, while I struggle to keep a steady grasp on Bodhi so he doesn't hit his head on the cement. "I want to go to McDonald's!" she shouts, ready to bolt this time, with or without Scarlet.

"I have an idea!"

"What?" Jani stops in her tracks.

"Dr. Howe's office is just ten minutes away. Let's go there first to show her both of you for five minutes and leave. Then I can drop you and Scarlet off at the mall and take Bodhi home. He can stay with your dad and I'll come back to get you."

"Okay," Jani agrees. Scarlet helps me get Bodhi back into the car and we have a relatively quiet drive from Burbank to Glendale. And this...is a miracle.

*   *   *

It's a full house at Dr. Howe's office but at least we made it in one piece. Now I know why our appointment times are 2:30 and 2:45: a lot fewer people are here then. Now, every seat is taken so I rush over to the receptionist and explain the situation.

"We have an appointment with Dr. Howe at 2:30 and 2:45 for both Jani and Bodhi, but we're not going to make it then so can we just see her really quick for five minutes?"

"Hold on," the receptionist tells me.

"Susan," Scarlet's voice is panicked. Bodhi is slipping away from her, but at least she has him for the moment.

"I know. I'm coming," I tell her, looking over the room to find a safe place to keep him restrained until Dr. Howe comes out.

Two glass coffee tables divide the room so it's clear which group of psychiatrists a patient is here to see. "We need Dr. Howe," I call over to the receptionist in a more urgent tone, dropping to the carpet below her window, where Bodhi has now escalated to flailing around.

More time elapses and it's getting harder to keep Bodhi in one place. He somehow manages to bring his head alongside his arm and bite down, leaving an x-ray of his teeth on his forearm.

"We need to see Dr. Howe!" Scarlet shouts to the receptionist. "This is an emergency!" She looks at the receptionist like she's a piece of shit and I second that.

The receptionist comes out with a cup of water, but Bodhi's too far gone and bats it away. Scarlet and I maintain our stronghold, thinking the same thing. *This woman is nuts.* My eyes float over the crowd of patients, watching, waiting for their own appointments. It's been way longer than five minutes and Bodhi is still thrashing around.

The Office Manager comes out next, her wig-like blonde hair sitting like a crown on top of her head. "You need to take this outside."

"What?!" My eyes lock into hers. "You want me...to take my

son…out into the lobby…that has a hard floor? He could crack his head! This is a PSYCHIATRIST'S OFFICE and he's on the WRONG MEDS!!!"

She looks over the audience of psych patients, rolling their eyes in disbelief then walks back to the door that buzzes open for her then re-locks itself behind her last footstep. It's not like this is a library or even a grocery store, for God's sake. It's a psychiatrist's office!

"Can you just get Dr. Howe out here for five minutes?!" I shout up at the receptionist. Scarlet and I are losing our control hold over Bodhi. Both of us are getting bitten in the process. "He's not on the right medication!"

No answer.

Bodhi gives us a breather and Scarlet goes up to the counter, giving a direct order this time. "Please call 911. This is an emergency." Scarlet and I match Bodhi's wild moves as we lift him up, keeping him tucked in between two soft seat cushions, now vacated on Dr. Howe's side of the room. We're still struggling with him when a Glendale Policeman walks through the door, his hands rustling his gun holster as he approaches us. "Can I help you?"

"Yes. You can get the paramedics," Scarlet tells him, as I hold my breath. *Can't he see what's happening here?*

The Office Manager calls the Policeman over to the receptionist window. "Dr. Howe needs to speak with you." The Policeman is admitted through the locked door.

"What was that all about?" Scarlet sounds as creeped out about the situation as I feel.

"I don't know. If she can see him then why can't she see us?"

"I want to go…," Jani whines then stops herself. "But we can't… because of Bodhi." I'm so grateful for her ability to rationalize the situation. Jani has a profound understanding of what is happening here. And, she's on the right medication.

*   *   *

We're still grappling with Bodhi when the Policeman comes back out. "So, what did Dr. Howe say?" I try to gauge exactly what's going on here.

"She said he's having a manic episode and we should transport him to the nearest hospital."

Scarlet and I stare at each other, thinking the same thing... so I just blurt it out. "Why isn't she coming out to see him?"

There's no time for him to answer because the paramedics have finally arrived. "Who's the mother?" Their eyes dart between Scarlet and me, like one of us committed a crime.

"I am."

"Do you want to hold him? We can put you in a wheelchair. We're just going next door to Glendale Adventist Hospital."

"Yes. I'll hold him." He starts to calm down a bit so I'm able to put him in my lap, riding backward into the ambulance. I've never been to this hospital before, but at least it is a hospital. I was starting to fear they might take us to BHC Alhambra, where Dr. Howe told us to take Jani the first time.

"Scarlet, can you walk over with Jani and just stay in the emergency room while I go with Bodhi? I'm going to have to call Michael."

"Sure," she says.

I feel guilty dragging her into all of this. I know she's always saying we're like family, but this is emotionally and physically draining. And even worse, I'm going to have to wake Michael up from the deep sleep I promised him.

*   *   *

As soon as we're situated in a room, I call Michael.

"Doe?" he grumbles, half-awake.

"Doe," I need you to come to Glendale Adventist Hospital. Bodhi went into it again...at Dr. Howe's office...and the paramedics transported us here."

"Where's Scarlet?"

"She's in the emergency room with Jani. I don't know how much longer Jani will be able to stay. I know I promised you could sleep in, but we're going to have to switch out. Either you take Jani to the Burbank Mall or I'll have to."

"I'm coming right now."

*   *   *

I'm at the Burbank Mall watching Jani run around with a four-year-old girl in the play area. The little girl's mom and I are talking when Michael calls, frantic over the phone.

"What's going on?!" I'm desperate to know.

"Did you take Jani to her appointment with Dr. Howe?"

"No. Why would I do that? She's at the mall having a good time. Dr. Howe knows what we went through. We were in her office."

"She's calling me now and says she wants to see Jani."

"We have to cancel. I'm not going to drag Jani there again. She's playing with a friend here and having fun."

"Well, I'm still here with Bodhi waiting for discharge. Dr. Hyde called and said there are no beds available so we're getting his meds and bringing him home."

My heart drops. A part of me would like him to be admitted to UCLA because the meds have stopped working again, but the other part of me is so tired of making that drive on the 405 freeway. "Okay, just bring him home and we'll meet you there."

CHAPTER 24

THERE ARE ALLEGATIONS AGAINST YOU

January 9th, 2014

After all our experiences with Jani and now Bodhi, whenever I hear hard knocking on our door, I expect it to be CPS. And this time, I'm not wrong. As I open the door in my nightgown, ready to meet their challenge, my PTSD from the first CPS visit when Jani's was at BHC Alhambra kicks in.

A petite Filipino woman stands before us with two deputies by her side. One is actually hiding on the other side of her like he's guarding against anyone that might attack from the hallway. I can't help but notice that the other one is really cute with dark brown hair and eyes. I'm distracted again, just like with Zach, but I have to focus on the issue at hand. I know we've done nothing wrong but I have my suspicions as to what this claim is about.

"There are allegations against you," the woman says with a thick accent I can barely understand. Of course there are. That is their standard first line. And why wouldn't there be? I'm beginning to think we're the only ones keeping CPS in business. But I have learned and even in my nightie, I have my flip-cam ready for these special occasions. Michael is half-asleep in his t-shirt and boxers but is also prepared.

"Are the allegations against me or Susan?" It's so sad that we know CPS lingo and procedures.

"Both of you," she stares us down. This may intimidate other families but this isn't our first CPS visit. We've gone through this so many times and just to get our kids the help they need, it's just ridiculous. So, I treat it as such.

Michael sees one officer, then the other comes out of hiding and stands on the other side of the CPS Queen. Apparently, he's done playing cops and robbers. "So, what are you going to do? Taser me?!" Michael argues back. Yikes! He doesn't usually get this upset, but it is 2 am and he just fell asleep. I, on the other hand, have been sleeping since 7 pm so I'm raring to go.

"Stop it." I caution him, conveying my handle on the situation, even though I'm still processing it myself. Lucky for me, I used to work overnight shifts. I can still bring myself awake quickly to start reporting and this is exactly what I do.

"Let's just get this over with." Michael shoots me an irritated look, easing up his posture. "Come on in," he gestures but they remain at the door as I film.

"Can I have your card?" I politely ask the woman. She gives it to me, as required. With knowledge comes power and I use it. "So, you're Nina," I say, reading her name out loud.

"Yes," she answers, her head down consulting her clipboard as she flips through papers pertaining to our case. I suspect we're just one of the homes she and her crew will wake up tonight.

"What are the allegations?" I maintain my calm, while Michael maintains his impatience.

"There are three. One is that you, Susan, have been overmedicating Body."

"It's Bodhi." They always pronounce his name wrong.

"Bo-dee," she corrects herself. "Two, you, Michael, left the hospital without being discharged. And three, you both not follow doctor's orders."

I'm so glad I'm catching all this on tape. "I did not overmedicate Bodhi. I've never overmedicated him. He's not on *enough* medication. That's why he went crazy in Dr. Howe's office yesterday."

"Why you come to doctor office early?" She speeds up her questioning.

"Our dog died last night…" I start off.

"Actually, it was the night before last…" Michael cuts me off and I respect his sarcasm.

"Yes, it was the night before. I wanted to let Michael sleep in because he was up so late. We had a friend over and she came with me to keep our daughter's routine."

"So why your daughter not in school?" Nina seems purposely perplexed, causing me to break into a nervous laugh.

"Because it's Winter Break! Kids are not in school. I went to Dr. Howe's office early because my son was having a meltdown and I knew he wasn't going to make it to their scheduled appointments at 2:30 and 2:45."

She takes a moment to look over her notes while the two sheriffs scan our home then check their cells to see what time it is. "What this…I read about medication and you overmedicating your son? Let me see medicine."

"Here, I'll get them." Michael goes into the kitchen, reaching for the medicine bottles, then bringing them out and setting them on my grandfather's red antique piano next to the door. My batteries are running low so this gives me time to reload the flip-cam. After all the allegations are addressed, I will begin my own interview with Nina.

"Here they are," Michael says, not losing his sarcastic tongue. "And as you can see the medication is still in them. If she was overmedicating him a lot less pills would be in here."

"This is crazy! Besides didn't they take his blood and urine at Glendale Adventist? That shows exactly how much medicine he's taken. Your answer is right there."

"Actually, they didn't," Michael says.

"Why not? They always do at Henry Mayo?"

"I don't know."

"Well, then they were negligent!" That makes me angry, but I have to stay calm, at least until they leave. Nina pushes the pill bottles back to Michael. Apparently, she's done with my end of the questioning and turns her attention to Michael.

"So, why you leave hospital without doctor orders?"

"I *didn't* leave the hospital without doctor's orders," Michael protests while I hold my camera steady on her faceless expression.

"It says here, you leave without doctor's orders."

"Well, I didn't." Michael is arguing with her.

"Why it say here that you did."

"I don't know, but I can find the discharge papers." He turns to me. "You know, this is all because I didn't have the $50 dollars to pay the bill. The doctor saw him and said he was fine to go." I hope Michael will just pull out the papers and get this over with. These people don't care that Bodhi may wake up at any moment and if he does, that's the end of my sleep and Michael's.

Michael searches his med bag. He used to carry all the pills around in a plastic bag, but when we were pulled over by the police for speeding, the officer saw them in a plastic bag and asked suspiciously, "What's this?" We were on our way to Dr. Howe's at the time and I said he could follow us there and she would explain. He believed us and let us continue with just the speeding ticket. That's when I decided to buy a small computer bag for Michael to carry the meds around in.

Nina turns back to me. "There's a bite mark."

"Yes, because he bit himself," I say.

"Why he bite himself?" Her questions speed up again.

"Because he's autistic," I answer, my camera still recording. "Ya know," I challenge her, "I have behavioral services coming at 6 am. You're more than welcome to stay."

At this point, the cute sheriff takes out his cell to check the time again. I'm glad I am wearing my cute nightie. "What time is it?"

"About 2:30," Sheriff Cutie answers, shifting his stance to put it back in his pocket. What the hell am I thinking? Trying to be sexy in front of this very cute police officer while being interrogated for child abuse...again!

"I can't find them," Michael's frustration is only tempered by his lack of sleep. "Wait a minute. Scarlet was with me! Maybe she has them? I'll call her!"

"Are you sure she's up now?"

"Yeah, she's always up in the middle of the night. You know she has insomnia."

Nina continues with me. "You have names and numbers?"

"Yes, I do." I am searching my cell when Michael interrupts me.

"Scarlet doesn't have them either. I have to check the car." He motions to the deputies. "You want to come down with me?" It's not like we don't know one of them will be accompanying Michael anyway.

"Sure." The 'lookout' follows Michael downstairs, leaving me alone with Nina and the cute officer holding back a yawn.

She hands me a pamphlet with all the names and phone numbers of the so-called "resources" that I *know* she knows *nothing* about. "So, if you have services, why he keep biting himself?"

"Because he's autistic with intermittent explosive disorder," I question her knowledge. "Do you even know anything about mentally ill and autistic kids?"

"Yes," she looks down and speaks softly. "I see it every day." Uh, yeah. Right.

Michael comes back upstairs as Nina's phone starts ringing. "I can't find them. But they have to be at the hospital." I can't believe this is happening.

"That's true. They would have to be at the hospital," I put her on the spot.

"Can you wait a minute? I need to speak with my supervisor."

"Okay." I look over at Michael and the deputies who are rolling their eyes, checking the time on their cells again. "You guys are welcome to stay until our behaviorists arrive at 6 am. You can talk to them yourselves." Their eyes widen. I don't think they want to stand here much longer.

Nina returns. "So, why you not follow doctor's orders?"

"I *did* follow doctor's orders!" Michael shakes his head, frustrated. I've analyzed CPS tactics from our past visits. They speed up their questioning, repeating the questions to trip up liars. Of course, we're not lying but it's really sad that I know their script.

"It says here, you not follow doctor's orders."

"Here, let me try to get Dr. Hyde on the phone." Once, when I was in the hospital and paged him, he called me back from his private cell and I'd kept the number in my phone ever since. Michael and I are both in shock when he actually answers.

"Hello, Dr. Hyde, it's Susan and Michael Schofield. We have CPS at the door right now saying we didn't follow your orders today." I offer her the phone.

"Are you doctor of Bo-dee Schofield?"

"Yes," he says. How odd is it that everyone is awake at 2:30 in the morning?

She looks confused. "He bite himself."

"Yes, autistic kids get agitated and bite themselves."

"Mr. Schofield say he talk to you before discharge. Did he talk to you?"

"Yes, he did."

She shuffles more papers around. "He has bite mark. Should he not be in hospital?"

"He's autistic. Autistic kids have tantrums and bite themselves."

"So what you suggest parents do?"

"Is he sleeping?"

"Yes."

"Then I don't suggest they do anything."

"And *that's* what he told me twelve hours ago," Michael concludes his testimony.

"So, what would *you* do?" I press Nina, with my own interview.

"I would take doctor advice," Nina responds.

"Well, you're *talking to him*!"

"Thank you, Doctor," she finishes up with him.

"Thank you, Dr. Hyde," I say, ending the call as Michael shrugs and I stare at this woman, awaiting her next move.

She nods her head. "I follow up on this case." Michael and I just stand there, shaking our heads as she leads her posse away.

Then Michael turns to me and says, "You know, that woman drives a black Mercedes."

CHAPTER 25

GOOD HELP IS HARD TO FIND

May 3rd, 2014

It's been five months since Bodhi's last stay at UCLA. It wasn't long after our last CPS visit that he was admitted again and given Zyprexa. It's working but we have to raise the dose periodically to keep him manageable.

Since Zach joined the Army last month, our respite team has been so pitiful that when Michael tells me Scarlet is coming over, I breathe a sigh of relief. Right now, Scarlet, Michael, and Zach are the only people I trust to keep Bodhi alive when he's in the throes of madness. I can talk to her about anything and she just listens. She understands because she "knows crazy." She even confessed to me why she doesn't drive anymore.

"One day," she tells me, "I was sitting behind this car. We were at a complete stop when something came over me," her eyes well up, recalling. "I put my foot on the accelerator and just...slammed into it."

"Oh, my God." This strikes me with how powerful delusional thinking can be. "And no one would've even suspected because it was like a regular rear-ender."

"That's why I don't trust myself to drive. I take Access every-where. It's free for people with disabilities. The only problem is that they don't operate at night." A frown masks her face, begging for my hug. It must be so hard for Scarlet and Jani to live in this world. Possibly Bodhi too.

"We're going to lay out by the pool today," I lighten the mo-ment.

"That's what Michael told me so I brought my swimsuit," she says, taking it out of her bag. "You mind if I change in the bath-room?"

"No, go ahead," I tell her as I put on my two-piece navy blue bi-kini. It isn't much to speak of, but when Scarlet comes out of the bathroom, jealousy comes over me. Her bikini perfectly accentuates the small curves of her figure. It's all white with red polka dots. I don't even like polka dots, but I must admit it looks good on her. "You look so cute in that! I feel fat standing next to you."

"You're not fat!" she laughs. Logically, I know this, but I'm no-where near as thin as she is.

*   *   *

Down at the pool, we all splash around with the kids. After a few minutes, I hop out and read my book, enjoying the beautiful weather and the breath of fresh air Scarlet taking my place allows. I'm drawn into Susannah Cahalan's memoir, *Brain on Fire*. She did a piece on Michael's book, *January First* in her New York Post col-umn. Now, I'm learning about her month spent in "psychosis" that turned out to be encephalitis.

There are similarities to what Bodhi goes through, but the dif-ference is that he's always going through an in and out phase, de-pending upon whether or not the medicine is working. People with encephalitis can be cured and people with autism don't go in and out of autism.

*   *   *

After dinner, Scarlet is about to help Jani wash her hair when I hear Jani say, "You can go now."

"Okay," Scarlet says, meekly.

"Jani, don't be rude." Sometimes, I just don't know why Jani says the things like this but it's *not* psychosis. This is just rude. "Sometimes, she just wants *me* to wash her hair," I apologize to Scarlet. Later, Scarlet and I both give Bodhi his bath then spin him to sleep in his chair while Michael takes Friday to the dog park.

"You can sleep over, if you want," I offer. "You have clothes here." I'd encouraged her to bring a set of clothes in case there was an emergency with Bodhi. That way, if we needed her, she would be here. Most of the time, Michael drives her home. Access isn't available at night and her sixty-five-year-old husband doesn't like to drive in the dark.

When Michael walks through the door with Friday, I jump up, excited. It's my own time now! I can take a warm bath and read before I go to sleep. Scarlet usually occupies herself on the computer or reads to Jani. She's the perfect roommate.

*   *   *

Around 8:30 or 9 pm, I hear them walk out the door as I drift off to sleep. This also gives Michael a chance to talk. He tells me that I used to linger on his every word, but I can't do that anymore. I know he and Scarlet have bonded over their similar experiences growing up with mentally ill mothers. I wish I could still give Michael my time and listen to him talk for hours but now all I want to do is rest, so I let Scarlet give him the attention he needs. Tonight, he comes home later than usual.

I wake up, hearing the door open, feeling more rested than usual so I pick up my phone to check the time. Oddly, it's past 3 am. "Is everything okay?" I call out to him.

"Yeah," Michael says, short of breath as he comes into our bedroom. "I just ran into some traffic. There are detours everywhere. I kept being detoured around. There must be something going on at

Cal Arts because there was a lot of traffic."

Since I've been resting, I would like to give him some attention. "Do you wanna...?" I look over at him.

"Nah, I just wanna go to sleep."

"Okay." I'm not one to turn down sleep. At least he's in a good mood.

*   *   *

Michael and I love Sundays because the next day is Monday, when Jani and Bodhi go back to school and we get our break. Weekends are so hard because we can't keep them busy enough. Downtime for both of them has to be filled with some sort of distraction. Even though Bodhi is only going for an hour a day, he's moving closer to what it took Jani nearly three years to do.

Since we don't have a lot of money, we rely on the beautiful pool and Jacuzzi in our complex, including today. I can't complain. This really is the good life. I'm in the middle of my book when Michael's phone beeps next to me. I look over at it on the side table then go back to reading my book.

His phone won't stop beeping and he's in the pool with the kids. Michael's always texting these days and it's annoying, but I do it too. I can't concentrate on what I'm reading with all the beeping, so I put my book down and fiddle around with his phone. I'm not good with technology. I can barely use my own iPhone so his Android is completely alien to me, but I'm finally able to bring up the text. *Cool! I did it!*

It's Scarlet. She says that last night was the best night of her life and she can't wait to see him on Wednesday. *Huh?* I flip up through the past texts. Michael wrote that it was the best night of his life since his children were born. Am I really reading what I think I'm reading? I squint in the bright sunlight.

My stomach's a bit queasy, but I read on and remain strong. I have to. I look over at him in the pool with the kids. He's happy and so are they. I start to oddly relish the moment. Even after reading all of this, I'm not sure how I feel. This isn't like the first time Michael cheated on me. Back in May 2008, it was a colleague at work.

* * *

Jani had just gotten out of the hospital and Bodhi was six months old. I didn't know if I was coming or going the night he came into our room and said we needed to talk. "Huh?" I couldn't keep my eyelids open.

"Can you please look at me?"

"Yes," I yawned. "What's wrong?"

"Us."

My eyes flashed open and I really looked at him for the first time in a long time, standing in front of me, still in his work clothes. "What are you talking about?"

"I'm talking about our marriage."

"Our daughter just got out of the psych ward," I half-laughed "and you're talking about our marriage?"

"I want to have an affair."

My heart leaped out of my chest. "What?! Our daughter *just* got out of the hospital and you're doing this?"

"I haven't actually done anything, yet."

"I can't believe you!" Michael never talked like this. It's like I was looking at a whole new person standing before me. "Who is it?"

"I work with her."

I ran through the possibilities. All the women he had mentioned before. "It's Kimber. Or Heather. Is it one of them?"

"No, it's not Kimber or Heather. You don't know her. Her name is Dahlia."

My body shifted into full waking mode. "You know that if you do this, you're opening a door here," I warned him.

"I know." He stared at me with sorry eyes.

"How long has this been going on?"

"Three weeks," he said, flatly.

"Three weeks!" I laughed. "Three weeks and you want to do

this?"

"We've never had passion in our marriage."

"Passion?" My laughter quickly turned to anger, then sadness. I glared into his eyes, trying to sort out everything in my head. *What did I do wrong?* "I know I haven't been there for you lately. I haven't been there for me."

"I'm not blaming you." Michael was so irritatingly sweet when he said this that it made me physically ill. "I don't want to lose this chance to have something I've never experienced before. I want to pursue this."

"Okay," I didn't know what to say next. "So, what do you want to do? Do you think you're in love with her?! You *do* know that in six months, you're going to look back and realize how *crazy* you are right now," my hurt came out in pure logic, "and it will be too late."

"Maybe," he acknowledged. "But we've never had the kind of passion I have with Dahlia. Haven't I earned this?"

"You've *earned* this?!" All the organs inside me shifted. I could not believe what I heard. "Okay. Tell this Dahlia woman that you've *earned* her. She'll *love* that! It will make her want you more!"

"I know you're upset." Michael remained eerily calm and I couldn't stop hating him even more for this. "I can't live the rest of my life missing out on the passion I feel with her."

"You know, if you had told me this a year ago, I would have been devastated. But today, it's okay. Really, it's fine. Have your affair. *We* just won't be intimate anymore. But it's important that we keep everything together. Bodhi would roll with the punches, but Jani would break and you know it." Michael nodded his agreement. "So, just feel free and do whatever you want."

"I'm sorry."

"I'm going to sleep now." I turned on my side, shivering, watching through the corner of my eye as he turned and walked out of our room.

*　　*　　*

With Scarlet, I feel a sense of power watching Michael while I think about what I'm going to do next. I can't say the suspicion didn't cross my mind because it did. This has been building, but I guess I didn't think it would go this far. Besides, how far did it really go? Michael has never actually gone all the way with another woman since we've been married, as far as I know. But what do I really know? It wasn't long before he and Dahlia split up and he came crying back to me. He said he scared her away by moving too fast and then...*he said* that *she said* he kissed like a 5th grader.

So, what makes me think this time is different? I guess I could pretend I don't know. It is so much easier having Scarlet's help with the kids and I trust that she'll give me the right help, but I'm still feeling a little weird about this whole situation. And then there's the bond she's built with Jani and Bodhi.

I figure out Michael's phone enough to get the nerve up to call her. She answers, drawing out a wistful, "Hiiyyyee."

"It's me," I answer, straightforwardly serious.

"Hi-uh," she gulps, her tone matching mine.

"I just want *you* to know that *I* know what is going on and" I take a long moment to breathe. "I'm okay with it."

"I'm so sorry," she says, seemingly shock-filled with grief.

"I would rather it be you because it would only be another woman anyway."

"Please don't be mad," she begs for mercy, ignoring what I said.

"It's okay. I'm okay. I've gone through this before." Bodhi's crying and I look up to see Michael calming him down. "I have to go now." As I end the call, they come out of the pool. Michael's bangs are flat over his forehead. He never wears bangs. This is an unusual look for him, but then again, everything is unusual to me. I don't even know him anymore. Maybe I never did? The first time I was more emotional, but now, practicality courses through my veins. Perhaps it's because my kids' lives are at stake this time.

"Who were you on the phone with?"

"Scarlet. I told her it was okay you two were having an affair."

"What?" Michael's taken off-guard. I suppose he expected me to find out at some point but clearly not this soon.

"I know you two made love last night." I take a chance, exaggerating.

"No, I didn't."

"Yes, you did." I pursue this line of questioning, still unsure of the details.

His face shows only annoyance. "How do you know?"

I swallow hard. "I just got off the phone with Scarlet and she told me," I keep a straight face.

"She told you we had sex?"

"Yes." God, I hope he denies this part and says he just kissed her like the last time with Dahlia, but instead he gets angry.

"It's none of your business."

"Uh," I half-laugh, "if you're having an affair, it's definitely my business. Besides, I told her it was okay. We just won't be intimate anymore. What's most important is that we keep our family together because Jani and Bodhi are doing well right now and both of them would go crazy, especially Jani."

"Why did you even call her?"

"Your phone kept beeping, so I read your text messages."

"You told her I was going to have an affair when I started my new job in downtown LA," he accuses me.

"Well, you probably will."

"You don't trust me! You've never trusted me after Dahlia."

"No, I don't." I face him head on. "This time is different anyway. You had sex with her. You didn't with Dahlia."

"So, what?"

I gulp the hard, painful air in my throat. "Yeah, so what."

"I don't want to talk about this anymore."

"Fine."

*   *   *

Later that night, Michael begs me like his life depends on it.

"Please, don't put this on Facebook." Our lives are an open book on Facebook. Michael thinks I share too much, but who else do I have to talk to? It's not like I can leave the kids to hang out with friends.

"I won't," I promise. It isn't to do him any favors, I just don't want to deal with the aftermath of announcing this to my Facebook friends, let alone the anti-psychiatry crowd that follows us like a mini TMZ. I don't even know what I feel at this point, other than trapped, just like I was back in 2008. Leaving Michael would disrupt Jani and Bodhi's life. And who would help me keep them going every day? Our marriage isn't about love anymore. It's about the kids.

I pop my nighttime meds, hoping sleep takes me away soon. I knew my house wasn't made of bricks but I didn't think the foundation was so weak. I can't say I'm shocked or as scared about the future as I was six years ago. Jani is doing well. Bodhi isn't great, but we're managing. I have hope that he will get better. Still, how can I raise two special needs kids on my own? Michael may be an asshole, but he is a good father and we've been 50/50 right from the start.

Then there's the issue of Scarlet being so much a part of our lives. She has been there for me when I needed her most, yet I can't accept moving forward with her in our lives. And what does moving forward really mean? Is she going to move in? I don't know why this bothers me so much. I mean, I do know why this is bothering me so much but I don't know what to do next.

CHAPTER 26

SCARLET'S LETTER

May 4th, 2014

Ugh. I can't sleep. I turn on my nightlight and bring out my computer to log onto Facebook. My mouth falls open when I see Scarlet's post on my wall. It's a bit jumbled but I know what it means. "Susan, I do care. Aww... thank you for calling me. I'm so sorry. I want to be part of the FAM. Forgiveness is the key. I love you. PLS don't be mad at me." This is a mess. I have no idea what to say. At least no one knows what she's sorry for because then I'd have to start explaining. "No worries...we're good," I reply, with a heart to each side. At this point, I just don't want to get into it. I don't even know what I'm going to do yet.

"You OK, Susan Schofield. Been a little worried," my friend Angie responds. *SHIT. Now people are going to be asking me what's wrong.* "Yes, Angie. I'm okay," I start typing and then my fingers take flight over the keyboard. "Michael and Scarlet have been close for a while now and consummated an affair. They have my blessing for their new relationship. I will not be intimate with Michael, but we will still carry on as we are because it is in the best interest of

Jani and Bodhi. I cannot meet the emotional needs that Michael deserves and I give them my blessing. We are not getting divorced because our kids would pay a hefty price. My kids always have and always will come first." There are more than 200 posts that follow this one, from all sides of the equation. I explain that there isn't anything I can do to make this right. I was beginning to trust him more, but now I can't trust anything he says.

Well, there, I did it and now I can go to sleep. It's a relief to get it all out but Michael will be pissed in the morning. I change my password on all the computers because once he wakes up and sees this, he will log into my account and erase everything I wrote.

Michael is up early. *He's never up this early.* I guess someone "special" called him. His eyes spit fire at mine. "You are *evil*! You said you weren't going to post on Facebook and you did and then you changed your password so I can't get in!"

I smile, feeling vindicated. For what, I don't really know. "Well, here's the deal. I honestly wasn't going to post anything but when I saw the post Scarlet put up on my wall and then Angie asking if I was okay, I decided that I needed to just put it out there."

"So what?!" He waves Scarlet's post off like it's nothing. *Like my feelings are nothing.*

"So call her. Tell her to take down her post and I'll take down mine."

Michael bites down hard on his lips. "I gotta take Friday out." He grabs Friday's leash, slamming the door behind him. I don't see Michael when he comes back because Bodhi is up early and we've already gone out for breakfast at Western Bagel. Jani comes out after her morning routine with the adaptive therapists we now call 'The Shower People.' "So, who's taking me to school this morning?"

"I am!" Michael walks out of the bathroom fully clothed. Space is tight in our apartment so most of our clothes are there, inside the kids' old green plastic bins from IKEA.

"I know you start your new job in downtown L.A. today, Michael. What time will you be back?"

"Probably by six."

"Are you going to read to me tonight?" Jani asks.

"Of course, I am," he promises, but the tension in his voice is hard to miss.

* * *

Minutes after they leave, I break down in front of Daria. I've grown so close to her while she's been working with Bodhi over the past year. I tell her everything and she's tearing up for me, making me cry even harder.

"What do I do? Scarlet has a relationship with Jani and Bodhi. I thought I could deal with her still coming here, but I can't. And she's supposed to come over on Wednesday!"

Daria inhales. "I don't know."

"I don't either." I look up at the cross Scarlet placed on our wall and ask God for help. I need to talk to someone else. My friend Pam contacted us around the same time Scarlet did, after seeing Jani's story, and I'm still in touch with Carrie, my former behaviorist.

Alysha, one of my newer behaviorists, comes with me, and we all meet Pam, Carrie, and Carrie's daughter at "We Rock the Spectrum," an indoor play area with specialized equipment. Basically, it's an indoor version of Shane's Inspiration, the park where we met Lynn and Bethanne when Bodhi was an infant and Jani needed help. This is what I would love the whole world to be: Accommodating special needs and designed so other kids could enjoy it, too.

While Alysha's playing with Bodhi, I talk with my friends. "I have no idea what I'm going to do. Michael's fine with Scarlet coming over on Wednesday, but I'm not comfortable with it."

Carrie shakes her head. "No way," she says vehemently, making me feel like I should never have entertained the idea in the first place.

Daria must have called Devon and told her what is going on because she calls. "Hi," she pauses. "I was wondering…would you be interested in a marriage counselor? We could get it approved through your insurance." She is a good team supervisor.

I don't have much respect for psychologists, especially marriage and family therapists who've never been married and don't have their own family. Too often, they see things in black or white, like the pages of the textbooks they've studied, yet they lack the 24/7 life experience. "Not really."

"We wanted to offer it to you because we know you're having a hard time and fighting in front of the kids."

"Yeah, well now we're not talking to each other at all."

"Just think about it." Devon presses me.

"Okay." I hang up, more frustrated than before. "We're being offered a marriage counselor," I tell my friends. Carrie gives a "why not" shrug. "We wouldn't have time to meet anyway." I shrug back and then it hits me. "Wait a minute! I've got it!!" I call Devon back and thank God she answers. "Can the marriage counselor come over on Wednesday morning?"

"I can find out." I wait for a few moments on the line and then the answer comes. "Yes. She can meet you on Wednesday."

"At our home?"

"Yes. Then you have to schedule a regular time at her office."

"Great!"

"I'm so glad you're happy about this," Devon says, understandably surprised.

"I'm very happy about this!" I end the call, looking at my two friends, mischievously. Carrie and Pam want to know details. "The marriage counselor is coming on Wednesday, which means Scarlet can't be here. It's a conflict of interest," I smile.

*   *   *

It's almost 6 o'clock when Jani storms out of her room. We've already made dinner. Alysha is our behaviorist helping me with Bodhi's bedtime routine, spinning him in his chair until he falls asleep. Jani can finally entertain herself with her DS, something she couldn't do when she was younger. We're up to about an hour a night now. "Where's Daddy?"

I told Alysha what happened this weekend so she's 'in the know' with what I tell Jani. "Daddy's stuck in traffic. Remember, he went to downtown L.A. for his new job."

"He promised he would read to me tonight."

"You know Daddy. He's always late. Once, before we were married, I showed up an hour late just to prove a point, but guess what happened?"

"What?"

"He was an hour and a *half* late! I was so mad, but more at myself because that's just the way he is and I chose to accept it. But nobody's perfect," I remind her. She's a preteen so she gets an attitude, sulks, and goes back into her room. I don't know whether he's really stuck in traffic or not, but it is the most logical explanation.

Alysha and I continue our conversation over the memoirs we've been exchanging with each other. I'm giving her *Brain on Fire* when I'm finished and she's giving me *First They Killed My Father: A Daughter of Cambodia Remembers*. Bodhi is nodding off under his blanket. An hour later, Bodhi is sleeping and Alysha is starting her notes on his behaviors during her session when Jani's door bursts open again. "Where's Daddy?" She doesn't wait for me to answer but instead looks over at the digital clock above the stove. "He promised he'd read to me."

"He should be home any minute."

"He's *never* coming home!" This is her typical over-dramatization but in this case, I'm not sure she's wrong. Michael was pretty upset when he left this morning. Could he have thrown all caution to the wind and gone to Scarlet's place, forgetting the time and the promise he made to Jani?

"Why don't we just call him?"

"Okay."

I call Michael and hand my phone to Jani when it starts ringing. She takes it from me, putting it close to her ear as she walks back into her bedroom. It continues to ring then goes to voicemail. "No answer," she says, handing it back to me.

"Oh-kay," my stomach turns. "Let's try again." I redial. His voicemail comes on and I get teary-eyed with fear. *Where is he?!* I gesture Jani to leave a message this time.

"Daddy, when are you coming home? Bye."

Alysha looks up from her notes. "Did you want me to stay longer?"

"Yeah, it would be great if you could stay a few more minutes." Bodhi's been asleep for a while now. Usually, Michael would be reading to Jani while I got ready for bed. Tonight, Alysha and I just stare at each other. I'm on edge like never before. Jani is doing this endless dance in and out of our apartment looking for Michael. Why hasn't he at least returned her call?

He could be stuck in traffic and his phone might be dying, but given what's been going on.... My mind travels to other scenarios. Scarlet has alcohol in her home. When Michael had an alcohol problem at sixteen, he went into a treatment center but he's been sober ever since. Could he be so far gone now that he's drunk, passed out on her floor? How do I explain this to Jani?

"Jani," I stop her coming out of her room again. "Do you want me to be honest with you?"

"Yes." Jani looks me in the eyes.

"I'm not sure when Daddy will be home. He and Scarlet are having an inappropriate relationship. He may have gone to be with her and lost track of time. I can read to you."

"I'm going to stay up all night and wait for him," she says, determined. Wow, no shock or surprise, just a solution. Not a good one, but.... What if the day she told Scarlet that "she could leave now" she knew what was going on?

"Daddy's breaking his promise. Does he love Scarlet more than me?"

"No! You and Bodhi are the most important people in his life. It's me he doesn't want to be with right now." Jani runs out of our apartment again. "I can read to you." I race after her as she runs to look over the balcony to see if Daddy's coming in. "You need to go to sleep. You have school tomorrow!"

At 7:45, nearly two hours after Jani started asking for him, Michael opens the door and I nearly pass out at the sight of him, his work clothes area mess and he never did call back. I thank Alysha for staying way past her shift as she walks out.

"Daddy!" Jani screams, happy at last.

"You're home?!" I don't even try to hide my surprise.

"Yeah, I'm home. I was stuck in traffic and my phone died."

"Oh." Whoops.

"Are you going to read to me?" Jani asks.

"Yes, of course I'm going to read to you." Michael moves past me to Jani's room, while I stay out in the living room thinking of how I'm going to explain to him what I just told Jani. She's not one to keep secrets very well. Then again, I guess I guess I'm not either.

*   *   *

When Michael closes the door to Jani's room, I just start into it. "I had to tell Jani what's been going on with you and Scarlet." This time, I'm wide awake. He looks at me, shocked. "She doesn't care," I say, hoping this will soften the blow. "She just wanted you home."

"You told her WHAT?!"

"I told her that you might be stuck in traffic or you might be at Scarlet's."

"Why would you do that?!"

"Because I didn't know where you were and you didn't call back! We kept calling and left a message for you."

"I told you. My phone died."

"Yeah, but you could have stopped somewhere and called."

"Maybe I didn't want to call you!" He acts like a snotty child.

"By the way, Scarlet can't come over on Wednesday."

"Why not?"

"Because our new marriage counselor is coming over Wednesday morning." I smile again, delighted with myself.

"A marriage counselor?" Michael's face freezes. He looks confused.

"It would be a conflict of interest for Scarlet to be here that day." I smile, leaving him with that thought as I mosey out of the room.

CHAPTER 27

DON'T FUCK WITH CRAZY

May 7th, 2014

Surprisingly, I actually like our new marriage counselor, Cynthia. She could be a friend. Better still, she's able to do the job I've intended for her. It's also comforting to have Devon at our table listening to Michael and I argue back and forth. The best part is that I get to text Scarlet and tell her that a marriage counselor is here so she can't come over. I can't say that I won't miss her help but I've concluded that I can't live with her in my home anymore.

"I need both of you to fill out the intake forms so we can officially start next week," Cynthia begins.

"Okay," I'm accommodating and sweet.

"I don't see how this is going to help." Michael's bitterness only makes him look like the "bad one" in the marriage.

"Here's my idea," I say, looking over my shoulder at Michael. "If you and Scarlet are still together a year from now, then we'll talk about a new arrangement with her, but until then I don't feel comfortable with her in our home." Devon and Cynthia look like they're watching a reality show, glued to Michael, awaiting his response.

"I agree," he says.

"Besides, you may want to get married… and even if you don't marry her, what if she gets pregnant?"

"I'm not getting married again!"

"But what if she gets pregnant?"

"She's not going to get pregnant." His defenses are up. "Look, I don't want to talk about this." The shock shows on our faces. We are women and know what other women are thinking even if men don't. "I have to take Jani to school now," he diverts the subject.

"Okay, and you're coming back at…"

"I'm coming straight home. There's nowhere I have to go," Michael says resentfully.

*　　*　　*

It's Friday afternoon and I'm driving Bodhi to his one-hour school session at Old Orchard when our red 2002 Saturn sedan starts dragging with a familiar bump…bump…slug…slug…. I barely make the right turn and glide into a parking lot on the corner of The Old Road and Stevenson Ranch Pkwy before it stops entirely. *Whew. I made it to the Marketplace.*

I hop out of the car and see that my right rear tire is shredded. Now I just have to hope that Bodhi will be okay while I call AAA and, of course, Michael. I hate relying on him, especially now, but I need him. Then it hits me, emotionally. I don't want to get divorced. I don't even want to be with anyone else. I just want to get my kids to a point where they can have the best possible future, and Michael and I can pick up where we left off. I want to take spontaneous trips to Vegas like we used to. I want what we used to have.

Michael is at a conference to help families with mentally ill and autistic kids navigate the public school system, a conference I wanted him to go to and I promised I wouldn't disturb him, as usual. "I hate to bother you, but…," I explain my predicament.

"I'm coming right now."

This is what I still love about Michael. He's always there when I need him most. When he gets to the Marketplace, we switch. I lift Bodhi out of the car and put him in our SUV, then we're off to school, leaving Michael to deal with the Saturn.

*   *   *

Later that night, before going to bed, I walk out to the living room. We no longer sleep together, so I take a moment to talk to Michael while he's typing on his computer. The kids are asleep and it's peaceful now. "Thank you for today."

"You're welcome." He softens. "You know, Adam at Country Auto told me that if you and Bodhi were on the freeway when the tire shredded like that, you both could have been killed." His eyes show fear, warmth, remorse.

"I do love you. You know that, right?"

"No. I don't know that." Now his eyes moisten too.

"Well, I do," I say as tears stream down my cheeks. I hate that I love him more when I'm about to lose him, but it's the truth.

"I wish you would tell me this," his shoulders sag, all defenses down as he starts to cry. "We need to have these talks."

"I know we do. I'm sorry. I'm just always so tired."

"I know you are. So am I." We wrap our arms around each other, sobbing until he comes up for air. "I'm supposed to see Scarlet tonight but I don't want to go."

"What are you going to do? You know she'll go crazy."

"She's already bought the condoms."

And then the answer comes to me. "I know what to do." I go over to the computer and log in to Facebook. Michael watches closely as I write my status update, telling my virtual family that we're working through our marital problems and repairing our marriage. Once I finish, I look over at him. "Now, it's your turn. She's still on both our pages."

Michael slowly begins to type words on the screen as if they were already compartmentalized inside his head just for this occasion. After he's done, his finger rises up then comes down hard on

191

the enter key. We look at each other, fearing her reaction, and we don't have long to wait. Within seconds, his phone is beeping. "It's her. She's asking me if I'm just doing this for Facebook or if I really mean it."

This is going to get ugly. Scarlet is mentally ill and she won't take it well. "The longer you let this go on, the worse it will get."

Beep. "You're coming, right?" she texts. He doesn't answer. The beeping escalates. "Hospital time," she writes and we can hear the panic coming through the texts.

"You know what she told me?" Michael sits with his knees up, his back against the wall. "She said that ever since she saw me on Oprah, she wanted me."

"Oh, God. So she planned this."

"Yeah." The reality sinks in for him. "Why was I so stupid?" He lets out a guttural cry and we get into bed together, crying in each other's arms until we both fall asleep.

*　　*　　*

It's 11 o'clock at night when we awake to banging on the door. It's so loud that we panic. "Someone's trying to break in!" My mind flashes back to when Scarlet told me about the time her ex-boyfriend broke up with her. She broke into his house and trashed the place. "It's her!"

Michael races out of bed and looks through the peephole. "I can't make out a face."

"Maybe she hired someone? Call 911 now!"

Michael gets on the phone as the intruder uses a blunt object to bust the door open. "I need the police. Someone is trying to break down our door!" Michael gives our address just as the door's ready to collapse down upon us. "What?" He is obviously perplexed.

"What's going on?!"

"Someone called the police on us?! It's them outside."

I nearly fall over in relief as Michael opens the door and we find two police officers, one with his hand around a flashlight, clearly the object being used to bang on our door.

"Please, step outside." We both step outside.

"Are you Susan Schofield?"

"Yes."

"Do you want to hurt yourself?"

I double over in a nervous laugh then come up for air. "No, but I think I know what this is all about. My husband had an affair and just broke it off," I begin as the officer takes out his notepad and starts asking me routine questions like my birthday. This kind of basic information is used to determine if a person is in their right state of mind. Sadly, I've gone through this so many times that I've become an expert.

"It's true," Michael confesses on the spot. "I had an affair and the woman I just broke it off with probably made the call." The officers relax their stance, take our statements, and turn around. They are leaving for tonight but this is far from over.

*   *   *

Scarlet won't stop calling and posting on Facebook. Her last text to me is "I'm destroying you and every aspect of your life." Her last phone message starts with, "Don't Fuck with Crazy..." I can't remember the rest because I shivered so much at the beginning. I thank God when respite care arrives for Jani and Bodhi in the morning. Michael is sleeping, so I sneak out to the sheriff's office and file a report.

"The first thing you need is a restraining order," Deputy Marquez tells me, her voice soft and compassionate. "My husband cheated on me too. I know how you feel."

I didn't know there were tears left in me, but it still hurts, so I just nod. "The problem is she's crazy!"

"We get this all the time," Deputy Marquez goes on, "but for us to do anything, she would need to be standing right across from you, with a weapon pointed at you, making a direct threat. Otherwise, there's nothing we can do." And there it is. The actual problem between the mental health care system and the prison system that gets people on both sides of schizophrenia killed every day.

I feel helpless as I leave. Maybe I should just let this go. It's over now, anyway. Michael really put me through the ringer, but he's still a good person and a good father to our kids. I am determined to do whatever I can to keep our family together.

CHAPTER 28

MAY DAY

Mother's Day 2014

Michael and Jani are sleeping but Bodhi is up at 7 am so I get him ready to go to Western Bagel, our hangout since we first moved here. Everybody there knows your name, kind of like "Cheers" without the alcohol.

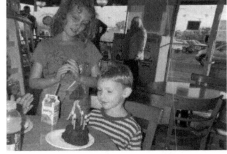

I'm driving out of our complex when a police car rolls up to the gated entrance. I get a queasy feeling in the pit of my stomach, as I see the officer shuffling papers to the side of him and fiddling with the entry code. I can't take it anymore, so I make a quick decision to roll down my window and call out to him. "By any chance are you looking for apartment 226?"

Jani and Bodhi on his 4ᵗʰ birthday.

He looks over at the sheet in front of him and I guess he finds what he's looking for because he gets excited. "Are you the one who made the call?"

"No," I sigh, "but I have a feeling I know what this is about."

"Are you, Susan?"

"Yes."

"Pull your car over right now," his tone changes like the wolf from *The Three Little Pigs*. If I don't do it, he's gonna huff and puff and blow my house down! I do what he says and pull into a future resident parking space in front of the leasing office.

Man, I knew she was crazy, but this is getting ridiculous. "I have a voicemail. I know what this is…."

"Don't…say…anything," his voice is cracking and his hands are shaking as he brings out his walkie-talkie. He must be a rookie. "Just get out of the car and put your hands on the vehicle." He fumbles around with his walkie-talkie. "I have the suspect detained." *Suspect detained?*

"Is this your son?" He looks over at Bodhi.

Bodhi says, "Policeman." Fortunately, and unfortunately, Bodhi's met so many in his short life. Happily, most at Western Bagel.

I walk over to the officer. "He's autistic."

"Ma'am, stand back by the car," he's getting really nervous now. He's gotta be new. I don't remember seeing him at the bagel place before. I do as he says. "Why isn't he in a car seat?" He wipes his forehead. "This isn't looking good." SHIT. We have one, but it's always tipping over and Bodhi doesn't like it, but I don't bother explaining as four other police cars pull up, surrounding us. I have no idea what she said or where this is going, but I'm scared—until they read the charges.

"We got a call that you're wasted and you're over-medicating your son with Benadryl."

I sigh in relief. "I don't drink alcohol because I don't like the taste and he's on doctor-prescribed medication." They watch me closely. "Can I take him out of the car now? We can go up to the apartment where my husband is."

I must not appear "wasted" since the officers' nod over at each other. One, probably higher ranking, gives me permission. I'm beginning to think that if Michael and I ever do get divorced, I should just marry a police officer. Life would be so much easier.

Bodhi is in a good mood and casually jumps out of the car, hopping along as he leads the policemen up to our apartment. It's obvious he's *not* over-medicated and by the time we get there, it doesn't take long for Michael to come awake and explain the situation. Again.

I'm shaking. My fingers can't stay still over the cell phone, but I manage to find Scarlet's voicemail so I can re-play her messages that explicitly warn me that she is going to keep calling the police on us. Then I show them all the Facebook posts. They exchange smirky glances. "So, what do we do now? She's probably going to do this again and I already talked to Deputy Marquez yesterday."

"She probably will, but all we can do is keep a paper trail going. And you'll need a restraining order." One of the officers turns his attention to Michael, pulling out a small pamphlet. "Here," he writes his name on it and hands it to Michael. "Take this to the San Fernando Courthouse and they can issue you one."

"Were you going to the bagel place?" One of the other officers comes out of the crowd.

"Yeah," I smile. I guess I didn't recognize him because he's usually sandwiched in between a group of deputies sharing tables at the back of the restaurant. He smiles back at me.

If nothing else, we're known in the community. Not to mention all the mandated reporters under the guise of behaviorists and respite workers in our home every day. Their job is two-fold. One is to teach special needs kids functional skills that their peers acquired more naturally through mimicking. The other is to make sure these kids are learning in a positive and productive environment where they're not being abused.

*   *   *

"Something's wrong here." Michael is typing frantically on his computer. "I can't get into my CSUN account." As he looks up at me, his panic-stricken face tells it all. We silently hope this is a computer glitch. Michael calls his work and is put on hold, but not for long. "I can't get into my account," he tells whoever's on the other end of the line.

There's a moment of silence as Michael processes what he is hearing. "I'm on hold again. They're connecting me with a Detective Archer." Michael's face morphs from anger to fear as he talks to the detective. "I can come down right now." He pauses to listen. "Okay, I'll come in tomorrow."

"Scarlet?" I ask like I don't already know.

"Yeah. She went to the English Department and gave a detailed report about how I supposedly raped her in my office."

"But you didn't bring her to your work."

"Yeah, I did," Michael confesses, making me realize that I don't know half of the story, but it's still hard to believe he raped her. She was way too willing and, frankly, way too tough. She may look like a Chihuahua, but when those little dogs go crazy, they go for the neck.

"When?"

"That Monday when I went downtown. I brought her there too. We even held hands, walked around. But here's the thing," his eyes grow big, "She paid for the motel. It was *her* credit card. The guy who checked us in also checked us out. It wasn't rape. And I never brought her to campus at night like she said I did."

My mind rewinds. "So, when you were late that night, you weren't really stuck in traffic?" That was the first time he *ever* put anyone else in front of Jani.

"No. You were right. I was with Scarlet." His body begins to crumble. "I'm so, so sorry for all of this. He wraps his arms around me as though I'm this treasure he didn't realize he had all these years. "I promise I will *never* do this again." He breaks into a scared sob. "I just want to get past all this and move forward."

I don't know why I feel bad for him in this moment. He's so sorry-looking but he brought this on himself. I really believe that after all that's happened, he will never do this again. Despite everything, Jani is doing well and at least Bodhi is better than last year.

* * *

Michael storms through our door like he's fighting a windblast. "They know I didn't do it!" He holds his Android phone up to God. "It turns out that the Google Tracker was on and tracked everywhere I went those days. It also showed that I wasn't where she said I was when the rape supposedly happened."

"Thank God!" We both feel a weight lift but the phone messages don't stop. She's not giving up. The restraining order is useless. At one point, after reporting that Michael raped her, she leaves another voicemail on his phone saying, "Let's just cut the BS and call me."

Part of me that is glad this is happening to him. If this doesn't stop him from fooling around with other women, nothing will.

CHAPTER 29

CURTAIN CALL

June 2014

I'm 44 now. Michael and I are comfortable with each other and he swears up and down that he'll never do this again. I believe him, but only because of all that Scarlet has put us through. The trust I had in him before Dahlia never completely came back. The broken bone healed but it still aches sometimes. I made it easy for him by allowing Scarlet into our home and our lives. At least, that's how I rationalize it. The truth is that she helped us during the hardest time in our lives, back when Bodhi was literally tearing up his own flesh.

If I weren't still young and healthy enough to want a physical relationship, I could just stand my ground and maintain a platonic relationship but I'm in need too. I don't want anyone else. Maybe Zach, but I'm too tired to even think about serving anyone else's needs, besides my children, and that would ruin any potential relationship so I might as well stay with Michael. I'm so conflicted. "You know," I say, contemplating telling him this, as he undresses in front of me.

"Yes…," he urges me on.

"I still can't get her phone message out of my mind."

"Which one?"

"The one where she says 'After all, we shared the same man.'"

He looks at me, helpless. "What do you want me to do?"

"I want you to get tested for everything. Who knows what she's been exposed to and that you could have exposed me to?" That's my final call. If he does it, I'll stay with him. If he doesn't, we'll just co-parent.

"I'll do it," he states firmly.

"Here's the deal," I tell him, wishing he had already been tested. "Once you've completed the tests and the results are in, we can be intimate again."

"Okay." He's like a child, ashamed of going after that piece of candy he really wanted but knew he wasn't supposed to have.

*   *   *

During all this chaos, Jani is about to graduate 6th grade. I'm so preoccupied that I don't realize her class is having an actual ceremony. Jani forgets to tell us that she will be going up on stage to receive her diploma. When we find out, I think about getting her a new dress but we find a fancy one she loves but only wore once in her closet. My mom bought it for her to celebrate her 10th birthday party and now, two years later, it fits even better. Jani is built like Michael. She has really long legs.

Her adaptive therapist arrives early on graduation day and takes pride in doing up Jani's hair into a beautiful French twist. The ceremony starts at 8:30. We have no choice but to bring Bodhi because one parent must be with the behaviorist at all times and neither one of us wants to miss this.

*   *   *

It's a thrilling sight for us. My daughter isn't out of place among her adolescent peers dressed in frilly formalwear and suits. Michael and I make sure to stand by the door nearest the exit in case Bodhi goes off. It's not long before we hear him crying outside. I hand the camera to Michael. "Just film!" Bodhi's separation anxiety has only grown worse over time but when I bring him inside the auditorium so I can watch, he wrestles around in my arms.

While the principal goes through opening ceremonies, I take Bodhi outside with his behaviorist and we walk him over to the swings on the playground. When I get back, Jani's getting restless too. Her fingers are riding through her braids, tugging at the edges. Bodhi is once again crying outside, but this time I'm relieved because it gives me a reason to escape. Which is worse, watching my inconsolable six-year-old boy with the built-in excuse of being little or seeing my inconsolable 6th grader look like a brat to the average eye in the audience?

I keep running back and forth, Michael filming as I anxiously pray that she'll make it on stage and I'll get to see it. Her one-to-one aide, Ms. Faith, stands behind her, a placid smile on her face as she tries to comfort Jani by patting her hair down, reassuring her that everything is fine. But Jani's not satisfied. She messes with her hair like flies are buzzing inside it. "It's itchy!" She screams as Bodhi wails outside.

I go back out to find our behaviorist barely able to contain him. I look down at the beautiful white tablecloth stained with red punch and a small slice of marble cake broken into bits on the ground. There's no time to react. I hear the names being called onto the stage so I dash back into the auditorium and watch Jani walking across the stage like any other 6th grader. No one would ever know what it took to get her to this place.

CHAPTER 30

FATHER'S DAY

June 22nd, 2014

Mom called to tell me that my grandmother took a bad fall and crushed her backbone. She's 97. It's close to Father's Day so I'm able to convince Michael to visit the Bay Area where she's in an assisted care home. Traveling is hard with kids but with special needs kids, 'hard' doesn't even begin to describe it. Airplanes are entirely out of the question because they would go crazy at the airport and what if something went wrong with the plane? We have to plan it out carefully, buying tons of CDs to entertain Jani and Bodhi along the drive. I sit in the backseat next to Bodhi while Jani rides in the passenger seat next to Michael. It's a relic from Bodhi's birth but for the reverse reason. Now we can't trust Bodhi.

When we arrive at her home, I get Bodhi to stand with Great-Grandma just long enough to take a photo. I stand off to the side and hold him in place. He looks like the most beautiful boy in the world, his freshly buzz-cut blond hair accentuating his blue eyes shining brightly. At least she gets to see her only great-grandson for possibly the last time. It's also a blessing that she can see Jani now.

At Bodhi's age, Jani was the one screaming, running all over the place. Now she still dances around but in one place so she can hold a conversation.

Our visit is less than 48 hours because Bodhi and Jani are ready to go. We came for one reason only and that was to see Great- 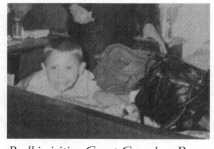 Grandma Rae. Mission complete. We pack up and hit the road again. Bodhi is getting antsy but we make it a couple hours before he starts to go off.

The 150-milligram pills only come in capsules, which he won't swallow, so his 300-milligram

Bodhi visiting Great-Grandma Rae.

tablets need cut in half to 150-milligrams. I am searching my purse for the pill cutter, but I can't find it. *It would be much easier if he would just swallow the capsule.* I'm running out of time. He's squirming out of his car seat and we're still three and a half hours from home. This is not good. I decide on the spot that this is the time so I pull out one of Jani's 150-milligram capsules and dangle his favorite Capri sun juice pack in front of him.

"Swallow the pill and you can have this juice." He looks at me and does it! Praise God! This is the very first time Bodhi swallows a pill and he doesn't go back, just like when I bribed Jani with a diaper. God works in mysterious ways. I'm just grateful he can finally take the capsules because life is a lot easier without a pill cutter.

*   *   *

Six hours later, we arrive home to find a middle-aged Hispanic lady with a round face in front of our door, an ID tag loosely hanging from her neck. It looks like she's only been waiting a few minutes. Perfect timing, I guess.

"It looks like you expected me." She seems a bit out of sorts, reading the matter-of-fact expression on my face.

"I always expect you. So what's the allegation this time?" I lead her inside as Michael lugs our suitcases up to the second floor, pausing for a moment to see who it is, then moving past her like she's a fly on the wall. Jani walks past her too, as does Bodhi, who runs up to his mattress and starts jumping on it.

"Well," she starts off, "there are accusations that you are over-medicating your son and that your husband's a raging alcoholic and an abusive father." I let out a spontaneous chuckle. I don't bother asking who made these claims.

"So, what do you want to know? The kids are here. Feel free to talk to them and look them over."

She nods and begins with Jani who is more than happy to give a tour of her room. She introduces her to our many rescued turtles while answering questions about if she sleeps alone in her own room. Jani is so familiar with CPS that it makes me wonder how many children are truly falling under the radar while we're investigated over and over again.

She tries to talk to Bodhi but doesn't have much luck. I had to put him back in a pull-up so he'd be more comfortable on the drive home. This makes it easy to show her that he doesn't have any bruises on him and is clearly not "over-medicated." We rehash the most recent set of events, even showing her some Facebook pages, and she heads out after a couple hours.

*   *   *

A few days later, we get a follow-up visit. This time it's a man with a computer. He interviews Jani who says, "There's no food in our house!" Besides bruises, this is *exactly* what they want to hear. She brings the concerned social worker over to the refrigerator and he opens it to find...plenty of food, just not the junk food Jani likes. "See!"

"Yeah." He sounds a bit disappointed. Maybe he'd like to see more junk food too? I tell him that he and his peeps at CPS or DCFS have become one big joke to us. He decides to take us off the "high-risk" list that's been in place since 2008. As he heads out the door he tells us, just to be safe, Michael needs to take a drug test and

I need to stop administering the medication to my son. We both stand there, shaking our heads.

Michael goes over to deadbolt the door after he leaves. "So, they want me, an abusive drunk, to give my son medication?" He gives a half-smile.

"I guess so." I laugh. It's good to find the humor in situations like this. But it does get me questioning the medications again. *Maybe my kids don't really need them?* So, as usual, I turn to Jani. "Jani, what do you think would happen if you went off your medication?"

"I'd be screaming all the time." Hmmm, not quite the answer I'd expected, but I really don't know what I expected to hear. Jani always seems to surprise me, so I go further.

"What about Bodhi?"

"Him too."

CHAPTER 31

A SCREAMER, HUH?

July 2014

Zyprexa has been Bodhi's miracle drug for over six months but, as usual, we hit the maximum dosage for a child his age and it stops working. It's the second week of July and Jani invites Bodhi to watch *The Lorax* in her room but Bodhi disappears into her closet of stuffed animals instead. Then I hear a sound I haven't heard in years. "Aah...aah...ahh." I call it the "schizophrenic scream," because it makes the short-aah sound like someone you didn't expect to see just surprised you, tapping you on the shoulder.

Jani did this at four-years-old. One time, we were at the bagel place. I don't know what set it off, but she just started that awful "aaah...aaah...aaah" scream. She couldn't stop, but as we walked out, a rugged, weather-beaten man in his late-forties was hanging around the chairs outside. His eyes, strikingly blue against his tan face, dug into Jani's eyes, then met mine. "A screamer, huh?"

"Yeah," I said, watching sadness creep into his smile.

A year later, I met a lanky fifteen-year-old girl with brown hair and freckles at Jani's first hospital stay in BHC Alhambra. She came up to me while we were going through the well-wishes Jani's first-grade teacher had the students send to her. "I know what your daughter has…." She's eager to tell me.

"Yeah?" I wait, anxious to hear.

"I have the high IQ too," she prefaces.

"Okay, so what is it?" Finally, I'm getting an answer. I'd rather it be from a doctor, but they don't seem to know anything.

"She has hallucinations. And you *can't* ignore them when you have them because if you do, they'll sneak up on you and go 'Boo!'"

Jani smiles at me. "See, Mommy! They get my imagination!"

My stomach falls to the floor. All I could remember in that moment was when Heidi Yellen, the psychologist who tested Jani's IQ at 146, told us, "She'll take you to places you never thought you would go." At the time, Michael and I were thinking math competitions, spelling bees, top colleges…. We never considered a mental hospital.

*   *   *

The medication is a little different, but the timeline is the same. Jani had a six-month reprieve as well. She was on Seroquel and Depakote from May to November 2008 when the meds had to be tweaked. Then, in the middle of January, the 16th to be exact, she fell apart completely, running wildly, pounding, kicking through doors and windows at her elementary school before she was transported to UCLA by the Psychiatric Emergency Team, otherwise known as the PET team.

Bodhi is relatively stable from January to July 2014. From what I've observed, his psychotic state starts with hallucinations then progresses to losing control over his body, like he's entered a dream state only to find himself caught up in a nightmare. Jani could tell us, "400 is awake. She's here." She could also say if she needed medication to put 400 back to sleep, but Bodhi can't communicate what he's seeing or hearing. Instead, he'll bang his fists together, harder and more rapidly, similar to Jani's clapping.

Jani has always seen numbers. I don't know if Bodhi does or not, but he uses numbers to categorize what he sees, like his bedroom is Castle Number 1, the bathroom is Castle Number 2, and the living room is Castle Number 3. This all sounds pretty harmless until his eyes circle around the room as he says, "I'm Humpty Dumpty." When Bodhi is Humpty Dumpty, he'll go to the refrigerator and get the eggs out and toss them, until their yolk splatters on the floor, then climb on top of the kitchen counter, crawling around until he has "a great fall." That's when he throws himself off the counter. Sometimes he'll laugh hysterically afterward and other times he'll cry, seemingly in shock at what just happened. In the earlier years, I just thought he couldn't tell me that he wanted scrambled eggs, but now we take him back to UCLA, again, when he's at this point.

After we visit Bodhi at the hospital, we stop at Starbucks. The three of us take our time, soaking up the peaceful air before crossing over to the parking garage. Five years ago, Michael and I were strolling back to this lot with our toddler, Bodhi. Today, we're with a young woman who is almost five feet tall. Michael turns to me, smiling. "This is cool. It's like we're walking with a friend, not a child."

I smile back at him. "I was thinking the same thing."

*   *   *

Jani successfully completed summer school and starts 7th grade in a couple weeks so we bring her to Bodhi's family meeting. She's almost twelve and determined to speak up for her brother. Before Clozaril, she was given a 50/50 prognosis, the same prognosis Bodhi is being given now. His discharge summaries have gone from "good" to "fair" in a year's time.

Before our round of introductions, Jani signs a release form, meaning she is no longer looked at as a child but as a young lady. "Jani Schofield...sister," she smiles with pride as we go around the table, then speaks directly to me. "I'm going to be a strong woman,

Mommy, because you're a strong woman." WOW.

There are no words I can say, other than, "I love you."

"I love you, too, Mommy." And this is the best reward I could ever receive. We continue the introductions with Dr. Emily asking what we've seen during our last visits with Bodhi.

"It's the usual. He's still self-harming. He has bruises and teeth marks up and down his arms and legs." Because the hospital treats this as "behavioral," he is always put into "time-outs" where his self-injuries worsen. I don't say this out loud because it is a given. "His thumb is completely swollen from him constantly chewing on it and his fingers are red from the chewing too."

They listen to our analysis, then Jani gives hers. "I would like to speak up for my brother," Jani begins. She's so serious. We all sit tight, eager to hear what she will say next. "I believe Bodhi would be helped by Clozaril and Thorazine."

"And why do you think this?" Dr. Emily asks her.

"I believe he has schizoaffective disorder (this is a psychosis resembling schizophrenia, but has periodic symptoms of mood or affective disorders), or schizophrenia. I've seen him hallucinate and then go into rages. He can't control it." We listen as she concludes her statement.

"You did a great job, Jani," I smile at her, my pride uncontainable. "Now, it's time for us to listen to Dr. Emily." And she does. Nothing any of us said changes the decisions on his medication but at least Jani was given the same respect we were. For whatever reason, they don't see what we do, but this is the process or "game" we all have to play out.

After a few days, Bodhi is discharged on the antipsychotic Geodon in place of Zyprexa. He is still on Lithium and so far, it's working "okay" but from what I can see, we're still only halfway there. We're still living on a prayer.

CHAPTER 32

THE SONG OF THE RIVER

August 2014

"I did it!" Jani runs up to me, her new fifty-something model-like aide walking leisurely behind. This was Jani's first day of junior high and we'd been anticipating it for years.

"She had a great day." Her new aide smiles sweetly as Jani and I hug each other. It's been such a long haul to get here. With all his accommodations in place and behaviorists inside his special education classroom, Bodhi also made it through an entire eight hour day. But by the following week, both of them are struggling in their new schools. We get reports back that Jani's throwing her lunchbox and running through the office screaming she has diarrhea, a tactile hallucination that hasn't gone away. The way she screams about it, you would think she has diarrhea multiple times every day when in reality it's only a few times a year.

After a couple weeks, Jani settles into her routine but it's far worse for Bodhi. He's back to throwing himself on the ground, hitting, kicking, and biting his behaviorists. By the end of August, Bodhi's back in UCLA.

*　　　*　　　*

Dr. Beta is on-call this weekend. He observes our family visit with Bodhi. He watches Jani run in and around the dayroom. She grabs onto the side of a metal food cart and rides it through the hallway. Then Bodhi hops onto the foot of the food cart like he's about to miss out on a ride at the amusement park. Dr. Beta doesn't use labels anymore. He just stares at them in awe. "It's amazing how they can both tolerate such high dosages of medication that others cannot."

Everyone knows Bodhi on the unit, just like they knew Jani. The maintenance crew loves him because their Union is fighting for a wage increase and Bodhi throws feces around during most of the outbursts, giving them more work to do. Sometimes, he's laughing hysterically and other times he's crying. It gets so bad that the nurses complain to the doctors because they're the ones who have to clean it up if maintenance doesn't. But that's not the worst of it. Bodhi's mental illness is predictably unpredictable, depending upon whether or not the medicine is working, like when he knocked out his baby tooth by banging into the bathtub's faucet.

Then there are the good times, the reminders that my child is still in there, like when he wanted me to bring him donuts. He's so excited to see the pink box that he opens it up and picks up a glazed one. "Do you want the glazed one, Mommy?"

He knows my favorite donut! I never even knew he paid attention. "Yes," I answer, hugging and kissing him all over, as he hands me the donut.

"I can't control it," he lowers his head, picking at the sprinkles on top of a pink donut.

"I know." I hug him close, caught up in this momentary conversation. I want more of these conversations, but they only come when the medicine is working. "Jani went through this too," is all I can say to comfort him. And I hope it does.

*　　　*　　　*

It's not long before Bodhi is released but we no longer have an outpatient psychiatrist. Dr. Howe sent us a letter, essentially dumping us. She will no longer see Bodhi or Jani because she feels betrayed that we don't tell her every time we take Bodhi to the hospital. She claims that we did not follow her treatment plan. It's not like I didn't see this coming but Michael calls her anyway, begging her to stay with us because of our long history.

She hangs up on him in mid-sentence. *Why am I not surprised?* Fortunately, Danielle connects us with a new outpatient psychiatrist, Dr. Cam in Agoura Hills. We make it through most of September and October before Bodhi's in the ER's back room again. We even make a trip to San Mateo to see Grandma Rae shortly before her death. It's less than forty-eight hours, but it's a lot for us. Her breathing is shallow and her words come out weak as she asks about the kids, then her last words to me are "Good night."

On November 10th, 2014, she took her last breath and, as I promised her twenty years ago, I am at her funeral to read *The Song of the River* by William Randolph Hearst. I study it in the days before, deciding which words and phrases she'd want me to bring to life. She told me, long ago, "The cycle of life is like a merry-go-round. As the old ones get off, the new ones get on."

*   *   *

When it is my turn to stand up on the podium to read the poem, Bodhi is wrestling in Michael's arms and I stretch out my hand to him, holding on tightly, as I deliver the prose as quickly, but emphatically, as I can. After I finish, Jani turns to me. "Can I say something?"

"No," Michael tells her, anxious to get off that pew as soon as possible.

"Yes, she can," I face him, stepping aside so Jani can speak into the microphone. She speaks so simply about how she knew her grandmother loved her. She was honest, sincere...pure. Then, as

213

we're scuttling quickly out of there, she surprises me once again with her incredible insight.

"They expected me to say something inappropriate, didn't they?"

I can't lie to her. I never lie to her. "Yes, they did, but you did great!"

"Yeah, Jani, you did!" Michael's pride overrides the anxiety he'd felt coming into the room. "In fact, you blew them away. Everyone, even Mommy, was so rehearsed, but then you came out and just said what was in your heart."

"It's true. It was beautiful," I hug her close to me.

Jani smiles. "We paid our respects to Grandma Rae."

"We paid our respects to Grandma Rae," I repeat as we tiptoe out against the side wall of the funeral home while Michael is losing his grip on Bodhi. Ironically, if Grandma Rae was alive she would be yelling, gruffly, at him: "Be quiet!" "Stop fidgeting!" But I have to believe that in her death, she realizes none of that ever mattered. What matters is that all of us made it here.

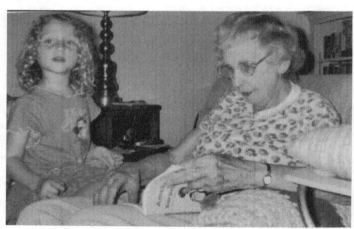

Jani with her Great-Grandma Rae in 2006.

CHAPTER 33

THE EMPEROR'S NEW CLOTHES

Fall 2014

Bodhi's losing touch with reality and I know it. It's a cycle and it's always the same. He stops eating and sleeping, and starts pacing in and out of his bedroom, trying desperately to get something to hold his attention but nothing works.

Whenever he talks about Humpty Dumpty, it's like 400 the Cat for Jani: the foreshock to the earthquake. It's only a matter of time. It could be today, tomorrow, next week, or even the week after, but the big one is coming and we have to prepare for it. I call our new psychiatrist, Dr. Cam, to schedule an emergency appointment.

While we're making the one-hour drive to his Agoura Hills office this time, I'm reminded of my trip to the zoo so many years ago. I have to keep my foot on the accelerator and move forward. He's already out of his seatbelt, jumping around from the back seat into the trunk of our SUV. I turn the radio louder to keep me distracted. Suddenly he's in the passenger seat! Even though he's right next to me, he may as well be a million miles away.

My arms remain stiff, steady on the wheel, eyes focused on each sign that shows we're closer to the exit we need. I pull into the parking lot, exhale my first sigh of relief, then get out of the car, take his hand in mine, and walk through the office door. We're in the safety zone, just an elevator ride to the second floor and we've made it.

Keeping with the routine, I hold him close to me as he wriggles around. This is not unusual for a child, especially a little boy, which gives us more leeway in the eyes of society. I'm numb to whatever he's doing beside me. I know he needs to use the bathroom, so I move quickly after handing over the co-pay, pushing the code to get in. This is a much smaller office, prissier, accented with mood-enhancing yellow and white paint that add to the bright sunlight coming in.

Inside the bathroom, I'm able to pull Bodhi's pants down and sit him on the potty. Within seconds, he tugs at his pant legs and pulls his pants entirely off. I hold him down on the potty seat, but he won't go. He looks down and sees the brown skid marks on his underwear, so he shucks them off. Then he lifts his shirt over his head, tossing it aside. He's completely naked, but I remain calm, trying desperately to get his clothes back on.

"Just wear your pants. You don't have to wear your underwear." I plead with him, but it's no use. He's twisting himself around me, to the point that I lose what little control I had over him. "Bodhi Schofield," I hear one of the receptionists behind the window call out but my voice is silent to the call.

I breathe in and out. I am calm in the middle of the storm.

I come out of the bathroom, with my naked son beside me, his soiled clothes in my hand. My only hope is that since this is a psychiatrist's office they will sympathize, unlike Dr. Howe's office, but their initial shock is hard to miss. Then they smile, shrug it off, and open the door, waving me back to Dr. Cam's office. I guess they've seen it all before.

I casually walk in to Dr. Cam, whose eyes widen at the sight of my six-year-old son ready to sit down on his nice white leather, or pleather, couch in his birthday suit.

"I can't see him like this!" Dr. Cam flails his arms around.

"I tried to get his clothes back on, but he won't let me. I think I should take him to the hospital."

"Yes! Take him right now and have them call me."

"Okay," I say, then walk my still-naked little boy back out to the lobby where there are two policemen coming up behind me. *Oh no, not again.* I close my eyes, hoping they'll just go away. And, I'm lucky. There not here for us. They'd come from another psychiatrist's office where a teenager was going off. As we ride down in the elevator together, one police officer mentions how, when he was a child, he used to love to run around naked too.

I smile, not in the mood to explain that this is way beyond a child wanting to run around naked. And if this same officer were to see Bodhi doing this even 5 years later, Bodhi would probably not be treated so kindly. Ultimately, this is what I'm up against. I have to find a way to connect the symptomatic behaviors of a neurological brain-based illness in a child to an adult's erratic behavior caused by the very same reason.

Right now, Bodhi associates the police with keeping him safe and my goal, along with so many other families with mentally ill and autistic kids, is to educate these officers so they'll recognize it when they see it. These kids are not going to be "cooperative" because they're living in two or more different worlds and cannot decipher which one is real, much like a nightmare where you can't control what you are doing, only to wake up and find the police beating on you, sometimes killing you in the process.

*   *   *

When I get back in the car, I put a blanket around Bodhi and give him two PRNs of Benadryl. He calms so much during the ride to UCLA that other than him coming in naked, they're wondering why we're here. Nonetheless, we were doctor-ordered to be here so they take us into an ER room but not the back ward.

A few minutes later, Bodhi realizes where he is and, dressed in his little white gown, steps out of the room, walking with purpose over to the two security guards, one sitting and the other leaning against the wall at the exit. "Can you get me back there?" Bodhi looks at the sitting guard who is eye level to him then turns and points to the room at the far end of the hall.

"Take you where?" The guard sits up, his eyes scrunched together, cracking a smile over at his partner in crime.

"Back there," Bodhi continues to point to the back ward, but the two officers just eye each other in a comical exchange, then look up at me, confused.

"He wants to go to the back, where the psychiatric patients are held before being admitted," I explain, knowing I must look ridiculous, especially since Bodhi sounds so rational in this moment. They laugh out loud and I'm not in the mood to lecture them on mental illness, so I just smile and lead Bodhi back to his room, telling him everything will be okay.

An hour or two, possibly three, pass by before Dr. Emily comes in. She heard that Bodhi is back in the ER and wanted to come visit him. He grabs her hand, begging, "Can you take me back up there?! We can read Dr. Seuss books!" He pleads, as she gently pulls her hand away.

"I'm not on that rotation anymore, but I'll see what I can do," she tells him.

"You were right to prescribe the Geodon. It's working!" I compliment her. "I just think he needs to go up on it. And Dr. Cam won't see him because he took off all his clothes at his office."

"I'll see what I can do," she smiles a straight line, her eyes showing defeat. It's a painfully heart-warming sight, but she just nonverbally told me that we'll have to wait for another "incident," one where he is a threat to himself or others, before he's admitted.

*   *   *

Michael, Jani, and I are trick-or-treating down the dark streets of an extravagantly decked out neighborhood. Tonight is the perfect temperature and we stop to take pictures at a pirate ship on some-one's driveway. Jani makes a beautiful Elsa, standing like a queen next to the new friends she's made through support groups, includ-ing our own Jani Foundation in the Santa Clarita Valley.

Support groups are great because none of us have to explain why our kids act the way they do. The best part is that we're capable of caring for each other's children. It's become our instinct. The kids must sense this because they're more relaxed too. They're not only loved for who they are but appreciated for their uniquenesses.

Meanwhile, Bodhi is at UCLA where the doctors are raising the Geodon from 80 to 100 milligrams. It is working on his behavior, slowing down his movements so he can focus and function in an everyday routine. But just as we're about to stop at another house, we get the call. Kevin, one of our most trusted nurses, is frantic over the phone, so much so that we can hear his own rapid heartbeat. "I just wanted to call...and first...tell you...." He takes another short breath, "that Bodhi is okay." This alone sends us into post-traumatic stress. Despite all the noise around us, we're straining to hear his words on the speaker. "He went into dystonia."

"Oh," I put my hand on my forehead, sighing in relief. "That's nothing. He just needs Benadryl or Cogentin," I tell him, as though I'm the doctor.

"Is he okay?" Michael asks. We've experienced this with Jani and know that it is easily treated and not fatal, but appears so much like a seizure or stroke that it makes you think it might be one.

Kevin is clearly shaken, replaying the event, giving us a clear pic-ture of what happened during those moments. It's more than pain-ful to hear about how he hit his head on the bathtub's faucet. Again, I remind myself that this could have been a far worse call. What this does tell us, though, is that he cannot go higher on the Geodon. They HAVE to go to Clozaril now. Clozaril has side effects too, but it is the medicine that is least likely to cause dystonia.

*   *   *

At our next family meeting, we find out that they are NOT go-

219

ing to try Clozaril, but instead authorize more Benadryl, up to 200 milligrams. And to think how many time CPS came to my door, accusing me of over-medicating him on Benadryl when I'd never given him anything close to that amount!

The very first time we met Dr. Hyde, we had no idea who he was until he introduced himself. He listened to our story about Jani, shook his head, repeating, "hard case", then walked away, continuing to shake his head. He treated Jani but says he doesn't see any clear signs of psychosis with Bodhi. Today, we see Dr. Hyde in the dayroom, dressed like he's going out to dinner after evening rounds, as usual. "Hopefully, we won't see you again for a while," Michael says as we leave.

Michael's tone is hopeful, but Hyde's eyes reveal a very different nonverbal message to me, shrugging off an, "Ehhh." He reads my expression, and follows up with, "He's definitely doing better." Translation: He'll be back.

*   *   *

By December 21st, Bodhi begins another set of odd behaviors. It's 6 am and he has his McDonald's breakfast in front of him while we eat at the bagel place. Even though Bodhi knows everyone who works here, he starts hiding from them. Few customers are coming in and out this early, allowing him the freedom to jump around while I unwrap his Sausage McMuffin and hash browns. I pour some ketchup on the side, luring him over to our small table. He begins to eat then looks up, staring out the window.

"I see Humpty Dumpty's ghost."

PART FOUR

CHAPTER 34

RING OF FIRE

January 2015

The last movie Michael and I watch together is *Walk the Line*. We'd both wanted to see it for years but never got the chance. We missed a lot of movies along the way. I guess I wanted to re-create our life from before we had kids. It was just us and Honey, who would "take one for the team" and let us eat popcorn and drink soda while we silently watched movies in bed all weekend.

But it isn't the same. There's no going back. Hearing the respite workers calling after Bodhi "you have to let your parents rest" is a clear reminder. They try coaxing him out of his own room, the one he shares with us. It's sad that he doesn't have a room to call his own, so we tell them it's okay. Since we can only afford a two-bedroom apartment, we gave Jani the master suite when she asked for it and kept Bodhi with us.

Michael never sleeps in here anymore. His back bothers him so he likes sleeping on the living room floor. I set up a TV in here so Bodhi can watch it when he is up at night and Michael and I watch on the weekends when we have respite. I smile painfully at Michael as the movie plays.

Johnny and his first wife are screaming at each other. She's busy with the kids and he's busy with his music. They're falling apart, and so are we. Michael's in his boxers and I'm in my lingerie. Our shoulders come so close I can feel how cold his skin is. My stomach rolls with the intense fight scenes until they come to a quiet end. But it's not over. Johnny and his wife continue to keep everything together until June Carter comes along. The heat in the air is undeniable, sending hot chills down my spine when he introduces his wife to June. I'm wondering what Michael is thinking now but I don't ask. He stays up most nights after I've gone to sleep, talking to "his women." It isn't just one, but I'm too tired to do anything more than make it to the next day. Sleep is my last refuge.

The movie climaxes when Johnny hits rock bottom, falling to the ground of his newly purchased home up in the wilderness. He's back on drugs and June comes to rescue him. She takes care of him like a baby, even going as far as to beat off a returning drug dealer with a baseball bat. Early on in our marriage, Michael told me he wanted a woman who would "go to bat" for him. I used to be that woman, defending him at every move, even my family's disapproval of our marriage. The kids are the ones I go to bat for now, even against him.

"Did you like the movie?" I turn to Michael, gripping the remote control in his hand.

"Yeah, I did." He doesn't look at me. He just stares blankly as the credits roll. "Did you?"

"Yeah, I thought it was great." I pick my computer up off the floor. I log on, refocusing my attention on the book I'm writing. Great movies, even not so great movies, inspire me creatively. I steady the computer on my lap.

"We're done, aren't we?"

"Yeah," I hear myself reply. It's more of a surprise to me than it is to him. I stare at the screen, blinking away unexpected tears. He picks himself up off my bed and slowly walks out to his sofa as my computer screen fogs up. I stop, allowing myself to sit with the shock of what just happened.

*   *   *

There's a familiar "tweety-bird" chirp on Michael's phone that night. I've been hearing it for a while now so it's become a rather annoying chirp. This one is Mia. They had an eight-month relationship before he moved to California. I walk out into the hallway and Michael stops me, his watery eyes doing a poetic dance. "It's true love." I shrug him off. How many times have I heard this one before?

"It's always true love," I 'Ha!' him. "Look, Bodhi's asleep so I'm going to bed soon, but I do have time to talk, even if it is about this nonsense."

"But you've gotta admit, we've never had passion before."

"I guess I just see us differently. I do love you."

"That's not what I'm talking about."

"Okay." I'm out of words at this point. "I envisioned our future getting better. The kids growing up. Bodhi's really hard right now, but Jani's improving to a point we'd never imagined possible."

"See, this is the problem. All you ever think about are the kids and our marriage has suffered because of it."

"I've been trying! Why do you think I keep fighting for good respite? You're the one who's giving up. Why do you think I've been getting all these movies for us?"

"Don't you get it?" He treats me like I'm his hardest student to reach in his lecture on love.

"Oh, I get it. You're always on the phone with Ginger, Mia, or whoever else you've got waiting in the wings."

"It's different with Mia. She was my relationship before you."

"And you LEFT her! You broke up with her..."

"I made a mistake."

I swallow hard. "I'm going to bed now." I know I should have expected this, but I didn't see this coming so fast. I have been reading Michael's texts to Mia and this time his voice is different. It's not Michael. The intellectual talk that once kept me hanging on his every word has been reduced to "lines" like, "You're my Angel" and "I can't wait to see you naked."

He showed me her picture last year before he friended her on Facebook. I warned him not to get started. But then, it's not like I don't have male friends I'm attracted to on Facebook either, so I let it go. Even before I found out about his affair with Scarlet, I must have suspected something either consciously, or subconsciously, because I showed Scarlet Mia's profile picture to make sure she knew that *she was not, nor ever would be, "special."* But Mia was his first real girlfriend. That makes it a little different.

Early on in our relationship, we used to share stories of our previous romances. Michael used to talk about the cross he wore around his neck that Mia had liked. He stopped wearing it years ago, but I don't remember when it happened. And we never did find, or even replace, our wedding rings after they disappeared when we moved back in together.

CHAPTER 35

ONE-WAY TICKET

Valentine's Day 2015

"There's a present for you, on the table. For Valentine's Day," I smile at Michael coming through the door. He looks over and laughs at the gift bag filled with Trojan condoms. "Just promise me you'll use them," I beg him.

"I promise," Michael is trying to appease me but I don't believe him. I worry because if he gets Mia pregnant and then "changes his mind," the consequences are irreversible.

*   *   *

When Jani and Bodhi are asleep and we're alone in the living room, I sit across from. His body lies against the black IKEA couch we bought so long ago, when we first had Jani. I took the cushions off of the old black couch and made it into a mini-bed. Michael and I may not be friends at this point, but at least we can talk to each other again. "What I want..." he starts, staring off into space like he's wishing upon a star.

"Yes..." because it is all about what HE wants.

"...is to have my own bachelor pad and for Mia to just come

down once a month." His eyes come down to Earth. "I really don't want to get married again."

I break into laughter. "She's not going to go for that."

"She's not like you." Michael is being snippy. "That's your problem. You think you know everything about everyone and you don't!"

"Okay, fine. I just need to know what *you* are going to do, so that I can plan around it. I need to keep the kids' lives stable."

"I don't know what I'm going to do," he says like an adolescent lacking the real-life experience he just went through this last decade.

"Okay," I sigh, then slowly retreat back to my bed, the only safe place I know.

*　　*　　*

Mia's flight arrives on Valentine's Day. I can't believe she's actually making this trip all the way from Minnesota to visit Michael. He's still married to me, no matter how bad things are. We're not even separated! In fairness to her, Michael is redefining our whole relationship, claiming we never had a real marriage. I guess that in this new version of our lives, she's not really fooling around with a married man.

I'm just rolling with the punches.

His shower is longer than usual, giving me time to satisfy my curiosity, scrolling through his phone, conveniently left on the counter. Michael writes, "I can't wait to see your naked body." Seriously? She texts back about how she's gained some weight over the past twenty years. He reassures her, "I will love your body. I'm sweating right now." I can practically feel the heat rolling off his phone. No wonder he's been in the shower for so long. Can't she see that he's going to fuck her, then come crying back to me?

*　　*　　*

Before he goes to pick her up at the airport we make "the deal." Again. We're going to co-parent the kids to keep the family intact. He will spend tonight through Wednesday at a motel close by and see how it goes. At least he'll be here for the kids during late afternoon so it won't disturb their schedules. I've warned him that she's going to try to get pregnant to keep him. He doesn't believe me, though. "Other women are not like you." He loves this line.

"So, other men are not like you then?" He sighs, knowing darn well that most of them are, they just don't act on it. Or at least some don't act on it. "Just use the condoms. You promise you'll use the condoms?" I beg him, again.

"Yes," he answers, like he's my teenage son instead of my cheating husband.

It all brings me back to November 19th, 2001, the night of Jani's conception, when I told him that "I never get pregnant" so he didn't need a condom. How did I know THAT would be the night I would get pregnant? It's not like we'd never done it without a condom before. But we planned Bodhi back in the spring of 2007.

*   *   *

"You're pregnant!" Michael stared at the stick in horror. I had just peed on it, handed it to Michael, jumped in the shower, and closed the curtain.

"What?!" I ripped the shower curtain open and faced him, my jaw dropping. "I am?!"

"YES!" Michael said this like a fire was burning and we had to get out now!

"I knew it! I told you!! Remember, the night after…? When I felt conception!?!?!"

"What are we going to do?"

"What do you mean, what are we going to do? We planned this, remember?" Maybe he forgot studying the ovulation calendar and making a special trip to Dr. Matz's to see if I was fertile? Sure, I told him it would probably take at least six months because I was 37, but we still planned it. How did I know I was THAT fertile?

"Yeah, but I thought it was going to take six months." He was breathing in oxygen but choking on the smoke still rising.

229

"What's going on?" Jani asked.

"You're going to have a brother or sister, Jani!"

"I want a sister," she told us, straight-faced.

"I know, but no matter what you won't be an only child anymore. I won't have to search everywhere for other children who 'get' your imagination!" Jani and I smiled at each other while Michael was suffocating.

*   *   *

My therapist is late. It's Wednesday morning. Since Saturday night, Michael has been living at a motel Mia paid for and now she's out of money. I actually made them peanut butter and jelly sandwiches to take back to their motel room when Wendy's declined her card but only because Michael assured me he wouldn't spend any of our money on her. There's only so far I will go.

I can't stop fidgeting with my cell, my fingers itching to call and find out how his "present" experience is going with his "past" love. I scroll down to "Mr. Doe," on my phone and take in a hard breath then exhale. *How did this all fall apart?* I hate that Michael keeps doing this to me, but I still need his help. There is no way I can be a single parent raising two special needs kids. At least Bodhi is back in the hospital. Besides, Michael isn't even sure he wants Mia.

I press the call button.

"Hello?" He doesn't answer my call with "Doe" anymore.

"Hey, it's me. So, when is she leaving?"

"I…" he stammers. "I…don't…know." Michael sounds like he's grinding his teeth.

"What do you mean, you don't know? Doesn't she have a shared custody agreement with her ex-boyfriend? You said she was staying until Wednesday before she had to go back to her daughter."

"She bought a one-way ticket," he grunts.

"Huh?" An unexpected chuckle escapes me. *For whatever reason, I find this funny. She is absolutely NUTS!* Dr. Ruth (not *that* Dr. Ruth) was right when she told Michael that all he's ever going to attract is psychotic women, so he might as well stay with me.

"I SAID...that she bought a one-way ticket." He sounds like he's blaming me now.

"So, when is she leaving?"

"I told you. I don't know." His temper's on the rise.

"You said she was paying for the motel. You can't afford to pay for...."

"She is! She just booked it through Wednesday night," he growls.

"But what about her daughter?"

"Her parents are taking care of her." My eyes stare up as Cynthia, our former marriage counselor turned my personal therapist, comes through the door, apologizing for being late.

"I've gotta go," I tell him, feeling momentary hope that maybe he'll be sorry for what he's done. Instead, I spend the next forty minutes crying, mostly because Cynthia's confiding in me about her own childhood and how her mother kept taking her cheating father back until, one day, she didn't. And that was the beginning of a better life for all of them.

* * *

The following day, I call Michael on his way back from work. I can't help wishing he'd just be done with this, again. I'm willing to accept an open marriage. I just don't want to upset the kids' routine.

"I don't know when she's going back!" Michael yells at me.

"What does that mean? Doesn't she have a daughter and shared custody?" I emphasize to him. He always told me how important it was that he be with a woman who put her kids first. And now he's doing the exact opposite?

"YES! But she doesn't have any money to get a return ticket. We already talked to her parents and they don't have any money either."

"What about her ex-boyfriend?"

"He's worse than you are. He's threatening her!"

"Well, you don't have the money either. You said she would pay for herself!"

"Look, I called my Dad and he's trying to wire me the money."

"So, what are you going to do tonight?"

"I don't know."

"She can't stay here."

"I know that!"

"So, where is she now?"

"I left her at the mall."

*   *   *

"He left her at the mall!" Melinda gasps over the phone. "He's such an ass!" Melinda is one of my best friends from high school and we've kept in touch over the years. She's been my hope and inspiration because she made it through a divorce, with three children, and since recovered. She even remarried and had another child.

The door flies open. "It's him. I gotta go." But I keep her on the line.

"You're late," Jani comes out of her room, scolding him for being tardy.

"I know. But I'm here now. I'm going to read to you."

"Okay." Jani easily forgives him, holding out her book, as he follows her into her room.

"Michael has added so much chaos to your life and it affects all of you." Melinda and I continue talking.

"Yeah, but he is driving back and forth to work in downtown L.A. At least he's coming back to read to Jani and take Friday out." In spite of everything, I still defend him.

"Then he goes back to Mia at night," she reminds me. "Think about what you're teaching Jani and Bodhi."

*   *   *

"He's coming out. Just stay on the phone with me." I'm admittedly a little scared right now and it's not of being a single parent. It's of him. His blue eyes are red, swollen...rabid. He's perspiring like he's coming off some sort of drug.

I break the silence. "So, what are you going to do now?"

"I don't know! I need money NOW!" He spits venom.

"I don't have any," I grab my purse, holding it close to my chest. He's frothing at the mouth. I've never seen him like this. I'm glad Melinda is on the phone listening.

"What's going on?" she asks.

"He wants money," I speak into the phone, watching him watch me, closely.

"Tell him that he needs to leave, now." Her voice is calmly pissed off.

"You need to leave now."

"No!" He shakes his head. "You can't kick me out of my own home."

"Yes, you can," Melinda responds on speaker. "Do you want me to call the cops?"

"I'm not sure. Just stay with me on the line." I'm shaking, but I don't know if it's from confusion or fear.

"I just need $30 dollars," he demands, his throat, scratchy. "We already booked her flight back."

"No," I say flat out, anger and resentment fueling my courage.

"I'm not leaving without the money!"

"Now I'm scared. Call the police, Melinda." The line goes dead in my hand.

"What are the police going to do?" Michael taunts me, his shirt dripping sweat. "I haven't done anything."

"It's a precautionary measure," I say as he glares into me.

Moments later, the police arrive and I tell them that I feel unsafe with Michael at home. They automatically look him over and gesture for him to put his hands up while they pat him down for weapons.

"So, what's the problem here?" A police officer turns his attention to me.

"We were just arguing," Michael says.

"You know we can't just come in here for a domestic dispute."

"I know that but he looked like he was about to get violent."

The police officers look at one another, then turn to Michael. "You know, sometimes after a bad argument, it is good for someone to leave the premises...to cool off."

Michael bites his lower lip. "Okay," he nods, relenting. "I'll go." They usher him out and I deadbolt the door, then get back on the phone with Melinda.

"It's not like he doesn't have a place to go," she says. "Remember, Mia is still waiting for him...at the *mall*!"

*   *   *

Our family meeting at UCLA is the next morning and the extra Klonopin I took isn't enough to calm my nerves. I have no idea what to expect. Is he here already? And what do I say?

"Is Michael coming?" Danielle asks, unlocking the door to the conference room. I draw a blank. I've never had to answer this question before. I always knew whether he was coming or going, or if he'd be on by phone, but now I don't know where he is at all.

"I don't know." Danielle stops for a moment and just looks at me. After knowing our whole life story, she genuinely seems as shocked as I am. I explain what's been going on over the past few months. None of this bodes well for Bodhi. This is an environmental stressor that they can once again use to refuse a Clozaril trial.

We're divided and conquered.

"So, he didn't call you?" I ask. "I would think he'd at least have left a message." He didn't and Danielle is as surprised as I am. This is out of character for Michael. Even when he doesn't like me, he's always in touch with the kids' doctors and caregivers. I gulp the air, my heart skipping beats. *I still love him. I still care about him. What if he's dead?* "I'll call him," I pull out my phone as we walk into the conference room, taking our seats around the table. It's just the three of us. The new female fellow resident assigned to Bodhi's case, Danielle, and me. I keep my phone on speaker.

"Hello," he answers, casually. And I was so worried about him.

"Are you coming to the meeting?"

"No. I'll have to do it by phone."

I can't help but ask, "Where are you?"

"In a motel."

"So, you got your Dad's money?"

"No. I called Dr. Ruth and she put us up in a motel for the night."

Another jarring laugh escapes me. "So, where's Mia?"

"She's right next to me." My jaw drops, and I look over at Danielle and the female fellow, both as stunned as I am.

Danielle brings us back on task. "All right, then. Let's start the meeting." I plant a fake smile on my face as I listen to their observations. Bodhi's medication is going to be slightly tweaked, but he won't receive a Clozaril trial because Dr. Hyde doesn't see any clear signs of psychosis. With everything going on, I'm too tired to fight. At the end of the meeting, I tap the End Call button, tearing up. "You handled that very well," Danielle praises me. I don't think she's ever seen me this vulnerable.

CHAPTER 36

DIRTY LITTLE SECRET

March 2015

"What am I? Your dirty little secret?" Mia's texts are getting nastier the closer we get to spring. She wants to meet Jani and I've told Michael that it's way too early.

"Susan isn't ready yet and I agree with her." I read his text back. YES! "You're so NOT treating me life a wife!" Mia screams her message back. WHAT? WIFE?! What the hell is he telling her now?! My thumbs on speed, scrolling up their messages as far as they'll go. Now, I can't seem to stop. I'm addicted. I'm at the ones I missed during the night….

"Would you leave my phone alone!" Michael startles me, coming out of the shower with a towel draped around his midsection.

"Why did you even leave it on the counter? You know I'm going to read your messages, especially when they keep popping up with that annoying tweety-bird ringtone. And she's NOT meeting Jani! I already let her meet Bodhi in the hospital!"

Michael ignores me, grabbing his phone back, pushing buttons. "There! I have a pin on it. So, YOU can't get in."

"Fine. She's not meeting Jani."

"I told her that."

"So, what are you going to do then?"

"She'll just have to deal with waiting until Jani's ready."

"Well...oh-kay," I back off. I guess I didn't hear the first bell ring when the fight was over.

"By the way, I did tell you that Mia's coming down again...." Ding. Ding. Round Two. "She misses me," he says like he's some sort of God that should be worshiped at all times.

Aside from Michael and me not being intimate, everything else has been pretty normal. Michael's been teaching all day, coming home at night, and reading to Jani. He even washes the dishes and vacuums. *And now she's coming back again?* "How can she keep affording these plane tickets?"

"She's not taking a plane. She's driving out this time. I told her I couldn't pay for a ticket so she left on Saturday. She's going to stay in a hostel in Marina del Rey."

I shake my head, trying to figure this all out. "They have hostels here? I thought that was a European thing."

"Me too." He shrugs. "She says she's really serious about finding a job."

"So, are you going to stay in the hostel with her?"

"No way! I'm not staying in a hostel!" He looks at me like I'm the crazy one for even suggesting this preposterous idea.

*   *   *

"What the hell is she thinking?! I swear I didn't even know hostels existed in southern California, or in the United States. I thought they were just in Europe," I tell Melinda over the phone.

"I thought so too."

"I know he's nervous because he woke up with colitis this morning. He thinks it's being brought on by stress."

"More like by lying in his own shit," she says, her sarcastic humor making me burst out laughing. Suddenly we're teenagers again, back in high school. "She's a Scorpio. She's not driving out here for nothing. She wants a commitment."

"That's fine but I don't want her meeting Jani yet. We just got through with Scarlet and now this? The only reason she wants to meet Jani is so she won't be kept as his 'dirty little secret.' He's treating me like *I'm* the mistress. She should *at least* know her place in all this *and* she said in her text that she feels 'so unmarried.'"

"She's delusional. She's *not* married! You don't know what he's even telling her. There's got to be more to this."

"At least he's seeing Dr. Ruth today. She can't possibly approve of what he's doing."

*　　*　　*

Since Michael's been seeing Mia after work, he's rarely home at night. I've taken over reading to Jani and she's restless in bed. She prefers Michael to me, but what can I do? "You know, I am trying to keep us all together," I tell her, secretly praying that he tires of her, like all the rest.

"I wish he were here to read with me, but he's with Mia." Jani pouts. She knows everything. We couldn't hide it from her if we tried. She's always listening in on our conversations.

"He's making a big mistake," I say, seriously upset.

"Daddy's making a big mistake," she repeats my own words back to me, sadness drowning out her anger.

"But right now," I catch my breath, "We just have to live with this. He's mentally ill and not on the right medication." I justify his actions not just for her but for me as well. I can't think beyond this moment.

"Maybe I should meet Mia?"

I gulp. Jani never ceases to amaze me. "Whenever you're ready."

"I'm not ready now." Whew! Neither am I. "But I know I'll have to meet her to stay close to Daddy."

I'm stumped. I have no idea how to answer this, so I don't. "Let's just read now," I say and she lifts the comforter over her shoulders. I knock around books in her nightstand until I find one of her Magic Puppy books where we read about Storm's latest adventure. He's hiding in *our* world, protecting himself from the evil Shadow lurking around, trying to kill him in *his* world.

*　　　*　　　*

"I broke up with Mia last night." Michael pops out of his pillowed- up comforter, holding his phone out to me so I can read the text.

Just when I think I'm past all his antics, I'm caught off-guard...again. So, I begin reading. *Oh, Thank God!* "What made you decide this?"

A long pause, then, "Dr. Ruth asked me to tell her what 'being in love feels like,' and I didn't have an answer." I nod. Finally, something makes sense here. "But that's not why I'm breaking up with her." He stares up at me.

"Oh-kay," I eagerly await more dramatic delivery.

"I'm breaking up with her...." Duh...duh...dummmm.... "...for her daughter." I'm so confused at this point. "She was going to give up custody to be with me."

What?! "She actually said that?"

"Yes!" Michael seems upset that I find it hard to believe she would give up custody of her child just to be with him. "She says she loves me. She's flying back to Minnesota to sort things out with her ex."

"But what about her car? Didn't she drive out here?"

"She's going to come back for it, eventually. She's just leaving it here for now."

*　　　*　　　*

"I don't get it," Melinda plays private investigator over the phone. "She's flying back to Minnesota but she's leaving her car at the airport? She's so stupid. Who paid for her ticket?"

"I guess she did."

"You really think so?" Melinda questions my naivety.

"You think Michael paid for her ticket?"

"Yes. How else would she be flying back? Remember, her card was declined at Wendy's."

I swallow the air. It feels different from what I've been consuming for all these years. "He's lied to me before, but he swore he wouldn't use our money to pay for her."

"Here's the thing," Melinda's so frank that it leaves me no room to debate, "She has to come back at some point because she left her car at the airport and that's going to cost money too."

*   *   *

I get off the phone and stomp into the living room where Michael's working on his computer. "You bought the ticket for her, didn't you?" I confront him. We rarely talk to each other anymore because we only we end up fighting, especially over Mia and money.

"What?" He looks up at me like he's trying to read my best poker face, marred by sadness.

"You said you weren't going to spend any money on her. It's *our* money!"

He curls his tongue around his cheek. "You spent money for Jani's new phone and didn't ask me," he counters. I nod agreement but keep a straight face. I'm actually getting quite good at this. I suppose it's a new, harder look but I can't afford any sign of weakness.

"I spend our money on our kids. *OUR KIDS*! Not another man!"

"I don't want to even talk to you anymore!" He gets up from his chair and grabs his cell phone. "Come on, Friday!" Friday follows him out, excited for his evening run.

*   *   *

I spend the rest of the night crying in bed until I hear Friday's paws paddling to his water bowl. Then there's the splashing sound of him lapping up the water in his bowl, satisfied after a good workout. I have no idea where to go from this point but I hear Michael's slow, calculated footsteps walking into my bedroom. He stands in front of me for a long, drawn out moment.

"I want a legal separation," he demands, flatly. I nod, my tears dried up, replaced by a stoic new mask. *Is this supposed to be a shock?* "And…" dramatic pause…"I'm intent on marrying Mia."

"I thought you just broke up with her?"

"I did. But she can't live without me. And I…I can't live without her."

"I understand." I keep my mask on tight but my insides are ready to explode into nervous laughter. He looks so serious. I guess he expects me to react like all the other times. Doesn't he realize that he's jaded me? The only way my body will respond to him now is with an involuntary laugh. Along with God and Melinda, my off-the-wall sense of humor is my saving grace.

*   *   *

Before Bodhi was born, I wanted to be a writer of young adult fiction so I read all the books I could find. One of the series I read was *Sisterhood of the Traveling Pants*. I buy Jani this movie and she watches it every day after school. Jani relates to Carmen, the writer who's emotionally working through her father leaving, marrying a divorced woman in another state, and being a more present father to his stepchildren than to his own daughter.

"I'm ready to meet Mia," Jani says like she's ready to hold a snake, the one reptile she's squeamish around.

"Okay," I say aloud, but I can't help thinking that I'm still not ready. "Then you call Daddy on your phone and tell him."

CHAPTER 37

A HOSTEL ENVIRONMENT

Spring 2015

The hospital released Bodhi but nothing has changed. I don't think UCLA takes us seriously anymore and Michael is working against me. He insists that Bodhi doesn't have schizophrenia, all of his problems are because he's severely autistic.

"It doesn't matter if he's severely autistic! Don't you see that he has ALL the ABA services he could possibly have? The behaviorists are with him all day at school. Taking notes!" I take a moment to breathe. "My point is that we are *treating* the autism, now UCLA needs to treat his mental illness."

"They're doing that!" Michael argues back. "Dr. Hyde sees 'no clear sign of psychosis.' What more do you want him to do?" I surrender. I'm so tired. I can't seem to get away from fighting wherever I go. Maybe it's me. Maybe I just need a break. Well, I know I need a break, but there's no way for me to get one without doing more damage to Jani and Bodhi.

Even with all of this going on between Michael and me, Jani is standing strong at school and Bodhi is better than he was last year. I know we're making progress. It's just frustrating because I know so much more than I did when we had Jani. It's like I'm re-watching a movie. Sure, I missed some things along the way but I still know the ending. I guess the problem is that no one likes a spoiler.

*   *   *

While Bodhi is at UCLA, a little girl in his class dies. Valencia is a small suburban bubble where everyone knows each other so the news spreads quickly. I hear it from a mother at Jani's friend's birthday party. Her daughter is also in Bodhi's class.

Everyone knew Evie. She was a bright and cheerful child who died in her sleep. Most of us don't know the exact cause but we knew she had health problems. The principal and staff decide it is better not to talk about it but keep her picture on the wall in remembrance. At her parents' wishes, a plaque with her name is placed in the school garden.

When Bodhi returns to class, he notices she is missing. Kids have always come and gone from his classrooms, even the other schools he's been in, but for whatever reason Bodhi picks up on the gravity of the situation. "First Humpty Dumpty, then Evie, now Bodh...AAAHHH!" He screams, fear masking his face as he points to an empty chair in our living room. Daria and Alysha are both with us and they go into full restraint mode. "UCLA!" He screams in panic. "I need to go to UCLA!"

I look helplessly at Daria. She's also been inside the classroom. "Are any of the other kids having this reaction?" She purses her lips together and shakes her head no, reading my frustration. I am reminded that my problems with Michael are minuscule in comparison. All that really matters is my children's well-being and Bodhi is unable to function in any environment.

*   *   *

It's been a long, hard day by the time Michael and Mia arrive to take Jani to the Castaic animal shelter. Daria and Alysha cup Bodhi's hands as I follow Jani's excited footsteps to meet her potential new step-mother. It turns out that Mia once wanted to become a veterinarian, just like Jani, which is a nice way for them to build a bond.

Bodhi's already met her so there's no shock in his eyes when he sees her again with Michael. She's rather reserved, an unthreatening blonde woman wearing little, if any, makeup. She's larger in stature than I'd previously thought. But Michael said throughout our marriage that he's always been attracted to Amazon women, like his mother.

She greets me with a friendly, guarded smile and we shake hands. I give her Jani's meds and look over at Michael as though I'm giving my son away to this woman.

*   *   *

"Mia got a job!" Michael shouts like he's just won the lotto. "It's in Marina del Rey, right near the hostel she's staying at."

"So, are you going to live with her in the hostel?" I love to pose my favorite question to him just to hear his response. He's already told me that there are twenty bunkbeds in a room and they all share a bathroom.

"I'M *NOT* living in a hostel?!" Once again, he looks at me like I'm the crazy one.

"But I thought this was *True Love?*"

"You know," he stares me down. "I really hate it when you mock me."

Like I care at this point. "What am I supposed to say?"

"You know what I really want? To just get my own apartment and be away from you!"

"I'll pack your bags." For the first time, I'm actually considering a divorce. Sure, I've talked to Melinda about this for over a month, even starting to plan the process in my head, opening up my own checking account, but I still lack the courage to go through with it. Plus, part of me still has hope and he is a huge part of Jani and Bodhi's life. The problem is that he keeps bringing more chaos into our lives when we need consistency.

*   *   *

A few days later, Michael tells me that Mia quit her job. He doesn't give any reason other than she misses her daughter and has to go back to Minnesota. And she's taking her car. "I'm living in Hell here!" I look at him, so done with being yelled at. We are right by the door when he points to the blue comforter he made into his own little bed. "And if I'm living in Hell, then YOU'RE going to live in Hell!"

I say nothing back. I remember what my Dad always said, "An empty house is better than a poor tenant." At this point, I'm no longer scared of being alone because I'm more frightened of being with him. Every step I take now is a step further away from Hell. Further away from my marriage.

*   *   *

My head and heart wage a war inside me as I wait to meet with the cheapest divorce attorney I could find. When he calls me into his office, we talk for a while. He informs me that about 90 percent of his clients are women. The husband wants out but for whatever reason, he doesn't file. It's the wife. In most cases, they say they're happier and wish they'd done it earlier.

God, I hope I'm doing the right thing. After I finish the initial filing, I can't face Michael, so I call him instead.

"Hey, what's up?"

His casual tone regenerates my courage. "Well, I did it."

"You did what."

"I filed for our divorce today."

"Wait…What? You really filed?"

"Yes. I really did."

I can read his mannerisms over the phone. I see him nodding, wonder in his eyes over what's next. "That's good" is all he says.

"Okay, so…that's it." I end the awkward conversation and my tears start flowing. Even though he's been begging for a divorce, like all those other husbands before him, he never actually filed.

*　　　*　　　*

When the day comes for him to move out, he's a bit teary-eyed, holding his suitcase up to me. "You really want to do this?" He found a cheap one-bedroom apartment, about 45 minutes away in Lancaster. It's $800 dollars a month. That sounds great for where we live in southern California, but he's not considering the gas he'll use commuting to and from downtown L.A and to see the kids. His misty eyes make me reconsider for a brief second, but I force my head to rule my heart.

"YOU want to do this!" I burst out. *Why is he always blaming me for decisions he's making?* "I didn't want any of this!"

"Okay!" He backs off like I'm the one dumping him. Then he just nods and slowly carries his suitcases down to his car, the old red Saturn we purchased a month before Jani was born in 2002. It was under my name but I just gave it to him. It's still running at over 200,000 miles and we decided that since I'm keeping the kids, I should have the 2004 silver Saturn Vue. It's more practical for a family and Michael is no longer a family man. Like Gerry Rafferty sings in *Baker Street*, Michael is a rolling stone.

The next day is a minimum day at Jani's school, but when I drive into the school's parking lot, I find her surrounded by her teacher, her aide, and the school psychologist, Ms. Felicia. I pull into a space, immediately rolling my window down. "What's going on?"

"She's banging her head against the wall." Ms. Felicia voice is calmly shaken.

"I wanna go!" Jani yells out to them and flies into the car, sitting in the back seat, banging her head on the soft cushion.

"You can't go like this. You're not safe," her psychologist tells her. Then I get a call from Bodhi's school. *I can't believe this!* Whenever a call comes in from either school, it's not good, so I just put the phone on speaker. "Hi, uh, Mrs. Schofield. Bodhi's been having accidents all day. Can you pick him up early?" His teacher asks.

"Hold on," I silently cry, passing the phone to Ms. Felicia. I have no idea what to say and I'm afraid whatever I do say will just piss everyone off, making *me* the problem.

"Hello, I'm Jani's psychologist and we're in crisis over here," Ms. Felicia speaks for me then hands the phone back.

"I can't come right now. Can you keep him there and I'll phone Michael?"

"It's okay," his teacher backs off a bit. "We'll keep him here."

I call Michael, hoping he can come. Even though we're going through a divorce, he is Jani and Bodhi's father. Whenever there's an emergency he always comes, no matter what. Can you pick Bodhi up from school today? Jani's struggling and we may have to go to the hospital."

"Huh?"

"Jani's been out of control, banging her head against the cement wall at school…"

"So, what do you want *me* to do?"

"Can you come and help out? At least pick up Bodhi? He's having a lot of accidents at school and they want me to pick him up early but I have Jani."

"I can't," he says. "I'm in Lancaster."

My jaw drops, "Uh…okay," I hang up, coming to the realization that I am truly alone in this. For whatever reason, I don't cry though. I just turn to Ms. Felicia. "Okay, so what would you like me to do now?"

"Jani," Ms. Felicia talks directly to her. "Are you going to be safe?" Jani opens the car door and runs out again. No one can seem to stop her. "Jani, come back! You're going to have to go to the hospital." I am frustrated with the situation. This is stress-induced psychosis, but she's still a threat to herself and others.

"No! I don't want to go to the hospital!" She runs back into the car and allows me to give her a PRN of Thorazine. Another few minutes go by and her anxiety lessens enough for us to get Bodhi. Jani calms more as we drive while I come to the very scary realization that our family is truly divided.

CHAPTER 38

WE CAN'T CONTROL THE WEATHER

June 2015

"It's sooooo hot in here," Jani whines. We're waiting in the school valet line to pick up Bodhi. The long wait is making it worse. Jani and Bodhi are fine with music in the car while we are in motion, but when the car is idle, their brains are on overdrive. "I have it," she whines, looking up at me, fearing the worst, "diarrhea."

"No, you don't have it."

"Yes, I do have it!"

I would say it's because of the heat but this happens every single day, even in colder weather. It's got to be a tactile hallucination. Really, this is the last part of her mental illness that we have to find a way to work through because it impairs her functioning. I just don't know how to do that yet. A Thorazine PRN only works for about twenty minutes.

"Then you need to go to the bathroom."

"No, I'll just sit here and poop all over the car."

"Okay," I sigh, inching up in the valet line.

"I'm getting out!" She muscles the car door open and runs to the nurse's office at Bodhi's school so she can use their bathroom then comes back a few minutes later. "I don't have it," she bursts back into the car. "I'm sorry." I have her apologize, but it has nothing to do with diarrhea. It has to do with her screaming about it.

We inch our way closer to picking up Bodhi, wiggling around in the arms of his teacher and behaviorist. I'm grateful he made it through the day. "It's okay," I pat her knee. Life is so hard for her even without the added stress of our marriage ending.

"I don't want to get divorced," she tells me, as though she's Michael's wife.

"Neither do I, but this is Daddy's choice. He wants to be with Mia. I can't control that. I can only control how I respond."

She sits next to me, staring out the window. "We can't control the weather and we can't control Daddy."

"You're right," I tell her, and repeat her very profound words back to her, for both of us to hear. "We can't control the weather and we can't control Daddy."

*　　*　　*

By mid-summer, Mia is back in Valencia and no one, including her, knows when she'll go back to Minnesota. I'm getting used to the idea of her being around. I even trust her more with Bodhi because she tells me the truth, like how Bodhi ran away from Michael in the mall parking lot and almost got hit by a car. Little things. Ya know?

Fourth of July brings us all closer, in a good way. We decide to spend the day together and go to the Valencia Town Center Mall. It's three on two. Three adults to two kids is actually quite relaxing. There are some positives to this situation, including the beautiful array of sparkling bolts of light spraying all around us.

It's Bodhi's first time staying up this late to enjoy the light show and it happens to be the best display any of us have seen in our lifetime. It's that beautiful. Large rainbow missiles thunder down around us, so fast and furious it's like the world we once knew is ending, leaving a fresh new one to explore in its place.

Michael holds Bodhi up high as he watches the colorful shooting stars parade around us. Once again, I think to myself, Bodhi's not bothered by the noise. Neither is Jani. Perhaps because he, like Jani, is seeing and hearing things all the time and this is just the more interesting sights and sounds momentarily capturing their attention.

Mia is good with the kids and I actually like her. She says she wants to move out to California, even show her mother the ocean. The only problem is that she can't move her daughter because of the custody agreement she has with her ex-boyfriend who doesn't want to leave Minnesota.

*   *   *

I make sure Jani's phone is on her nightstand just in case she wakes up early. She's thirteen now and can stay home alone. Friday stays with her, though.

UCLA never did solve Bodhi's sleep issue. It's close to 3 am and I give him his early morning meds, then take him for a drive. I feed him close to 500 calories, the only thing that makes the Geodon work, so he'll go back to sleep as soon as we get home instead of staying up all night. It's a different life without Michael, but I guess it's a life God prepared me for years ago when I worked all those overnight shifts.

*   *   *

Mia and I are getting closer. We spend a lot of time out by the pool talking about how she really wants to bring Lia to California. She wants Lia to have a playmate. However, Jani and Bodhi being Lia's playmates is only likely if she actually moves here. I still believe she wants another baby and that she wants this baby from Michael. I guess the positive from all of this is that Jani and Bodhi may get a half-brother, half-sister, or both, along with a step-sister. That's more people to potentially look after them when Michael and I are gone.

Then there's the other part of me. That part feels like Michael is abandoning us to start a new life with a new family and throwing us away. The tears behind my eyes are heavy. I know this is all for a reason, but it doesn't stop my stomach from turning in circles around my heart. I'm on my own now. I have two special needs kids whose future is anyone's guess and I'm going solo. I'm desperate for them to function.

*   *   *

The air outside is fresh, the sky, bright blue, and the mountains, peaceful. I love being at Central Bark. Mountains surround us and looking at them calms me, even if they don't take away my problems. Michael and I constantly fight over money.

"Hello?" Michael answers my call after I throw Friday one of the battered tennis balls he's found here at the dog park. He used to be the one who took Friday out every night but he's neglecting his duties there too.

"I need you off my Sprint account." I am calm, matter-of-fact.

"I know," he answers softly, like he really cares about me. "I can meet you at Sprint now if you want?"

I'm in pain again, emotional pain. I don't want to get divorced, but I don't know what else to do, so I just go through the motions. "Okay. Give me a few more minutes here with Friday and I'll meet you there." The Sprint store is just a few minutes away from the dog park and Michael is standing in front waiting for me. He seems distraught over all of this too.

"Bodhi had a really bad day yesterday," I say, getting out of my car. "He spent the entire day in restraints. They had to order black armbands, but even those weren't enough. Alysha had to put washcloths under the restraints to protect herself from his biting."

Michael is glued to his phone and doesn't seem as interested as I'd hoped he'd be but I go on. "So, I set up a protocol for the next time. If Bodhi is out of control for more than twenty minutes, they have to give him a PRN of Benadryl. If he keeps going for an hour, they have to call the paramedics, then me, and I will meet him at

Henry Mayo where we can request the Clozaril from Dr. Maki." Dr. Maki is Bodhi's newest psychiatrist since Dr. Cam backed out. "I can't just take him to the hospital anymore because they don't take me seriously. If it happens at school, they'll have to do something."

Michael turns to me, eyes distressed, as we walk into the store. "I just dropped Mia off at the airport. I was crying all the way there. I really do love her." He's weeping over her. Did he hear even one word I said about his son?

Mia's texts are coming in like wildfire and Michael is texting her back, his tears fighting off the blaze, reassuring her that everything will be okay. "Uh, you have to let her go now," I interrupt his watery stare, gesturing to the Sprint guy waiting on us. "You need to give him your phone to see if you qualify for your own account. I can't pay for you anymore. They're overcharging me as it is." My earlier good credit carried us a long way. Nearly everything from our cars to the phones is in my name.

Michael is approved and the guy hands his phone back. I glance over and notice my name is on his list but I'm no longer on there as "Little Doe Cell." Instead, I'm Susan Schofield. We have called each other Mr. Doe and Little Doe since before we had kids. I choke back tears riding up my throat. "Her boyfriend won't even let her see Lia."

I decide to keep out of this. "All I care about is that you don't go to Minnesota because Jani and Bodhi love you so much."

"I know they do. Besides, I can't move toe Minnesota. I don't even have enough money to give you." He turns serious. "I'm signing up with a temp agency."

"Can't Mia get another job?" He shakes his head. Apparently, this is the most ludicrous question he's ever heard. "Why not?"

"Because! She's living between two states!" His eyes are dead serious, so I work hard to hold back the nervous giggle breaking through my quiet eyes. At least I've got some great stuff when I talk to Melinda later.

*   *   *

"Mia can't get a job because, get this, she's living in two states!"

"She could do marketing," Melinda suggests. "How's Jani doing?"

"She's doing okay. It's Bodhi. His separation anxiety is really bad right now. And it's not just me anymore. It's his behaviorists too. He freaks out whenever there's a trade-off between them. He never used to do this."

"It's probably because he thinks it's his fault."

"What?"

"You should talk to him. Tell him it's not his fault."

"I know he understands."

"Of course he understands. That's why you need to talk to him like you do with Jani."

"I will," I promise her. "I just have to wait for the right time." *Once again, it's me who's not ready.*

CHAPTER 39

HOT POTATO

July 2015

"Are you sure you can handle Bodhi if I go down to my car for a minute?" *I don't think she really gets what I mean, but maybe I'm wrong?*

"Oh, yeah." This plumply sweet mother of two waves me off with a carefree smile. Sophia's soft brown eyes are comforting and she raised two girls to adulthood. So, who better, right? But then, Bodhi's not your average boy, although he looks like one right now, sitting with Sophia and playing with his toys. Then there's her daughter, Sylvia, who is here too. She's Jani's respite. Yes, there is rampant nepotism in the respite care business but since they're both here, I feel safe going down to my car to get more bottled water. The moment I get back, Sophia looks like she's just seen a ghost.

"What happened?!" I scan the room, looking for Bodhi. Jani is watching her TV show like usual, yet Sophia's daughter shares the same OMG look as her mom.

"He tried to jump off the balcony!" She shakes her head at me, in shock. "I've never seen anything like it!" Well, I have and so has

Jani. That's why she's still watching TV, unfazed. I look over at Bodhi and see that he's fine now, so I'm expressionless as I listen to her ramble on. Even Jani tunes her out. My pleas for trained respite have fallen upon deaf ears. I'm supposed to be able to leave during this time, but I don't dare do that. I was only gone for one minute. I don't want to imagine what would happen if I left for an entire hour. "In a split second" she begins again, the shock still on her face, nothing less than what you'd see on Yahoo News after a "bizarre incident" that only mental illness will later explain. "He went to the door to get you and then he came back into the room," she says, wiping her forehead, keeping her back against the closed balcony door as she slows her speech. "He put one leg over the rail. I got him just in time! It was a split second!" She reiterates like I don't understand what she said, even though I've been saying this all along and she didn't hear me.

"He did try to jump," Jani says, eyes fixed on the TV. She's as tired of the game as I am.

"So what should I do now?" I ask Sophia. After all, she is a mandated reporter. "I can't take him to the hospital because he's fine right now. Should I call 9-1-1?"

"Yes! I have to report it to my work too!" She sounds exasperated. For me, it's just part of the day and the reason I really can't trust anyone to watch Bodhi. He won't get the right help unless he hurts himself or others. I have to keep him as safe as possible until "that time" comes. I make the call and less than ten minutes later a couple of deputies arrive.

"My son's autistic," I say, pointing them over to Sophia. "She's my respite care worker who was taking care of him at the time…" I lead her into a story that, if had a bad ending, she would be the perfect "tease" on news channels throughout the nation.

She rehashes the incident and the police look over at Bodhi playfully jumping on the soft couch cushions. "I've never seen anything like it!" She catches her breath at the end of the story, like she's about to double over.

"I don't want to go to UCLA!" Bodhi cries out. And honestly, I don't want him to go either, but it's not my choice to make. So, I leave it up to the *experts*.

"It looks like you've got everything under control now, but we'll log it." Poor Sophia is still in a state of shock as the police walk out of our apartment. Jani is on the phone with Michael, re-telling the incident, but he is unfazed too. When he finds out that Bodhi is fine, he doesn't bother making the trip out from Lancaster. I sigh, comfortably numb.

I retrieve some duct-tape from the counter. I had wanted to give Bodhi some outside time, but I simply can't take that chance anymore. Melinda's right, I really need to talk to him about Daddy leaving. I just have no idea what to say.

CHAPTER 40

NAKED TRUTH

August 2015

On the way home from Wendy's, we hear "Flashback from the 90s." It's like old times. Michael is driving with Jani next to him in the passenger seat, and I'm in the backseat with Bodhi. Mia is still in Minnesota. "Remember this song, Mommy?" Michael asks like we're out on a family vacation.

I hear his words but I'm not really listening to whatever song is playing. Our life as we knew it is over so why does he keep trying to draw me back in? That's what it feels like. "I used to come into Shadow Traffic on the overnights when Mommy was reporting traffic on the radio," he tells the kids. "This song was always playing."

"Oh yeah," I say, half-remembering. When we get home, Michael goes off to read to Jani and I give Bodhi a bath and settle him down in his spinning chair until he falls asleep. It's getting late and I have no idea how long Bodhi will sleep.

It's dark and quiet in the living room so I undress to take my bath but, as always, I make sure to lock the door. Both Jani and Bodhi have a habit of barging in unannounced. I hear Jani's bedroom door squeak open and Michael leave. Soon after, it closes and I'm ready to come out and deadbolt the door. I do this automatically now because it makes me feel safer. "Oh!" I immediately run back into the bathroom. I thought you'd left already."

"No. I just finished reading to Jani." His jaw drops and I quickly cover up with the nearest towel I can find. I didn't realize how uncomfortable I would feel being naked around my soon-to-be-ex-husband.

"Uh, can you take Friday out one last time? I'm going to bed now."

"Okay," he agrees and I steady my towel, walking quickly into my bedroom and closing the door. I'm a bit shaky getting into bed, so I hold the covers up to my chest. Somehow I feel invaded, eagerly waiting for the outside door to open, and hear Friday's paws walk in and lap up the water in his bowl. Once I know he's gone, I can breathe again.

"Goodnight," Michael calls out from the door.

"Goodnight," I say, after hearing the door close. I peek out to make sure he's really gone, then walk out naked and deadbolt it. This is my home now and he's just a visitor in it.

*   *   *

The next night brings more surprises. After reading to Jani he comes in to have another 'serious talk.' *Oh God, these are getting so old.* "Mia has made her decision," he states like she's the judge in a family court. As usual, I'm riveted, so I listen intently for a decision that will clearly affect all of our lives. She is the judge after all. He waits a moment, to make sure he's got my full attention, then sits in Bodhi's spinning chair, inhaling a deep breath.

Oh, come on, already…. "She's going to stay in Minnesota with her daughter." *Of course she is, you dumbass.* "Now, it's up to me," he pauses, as the intensity builds around us.

"What are you going to do?" I am trying to make him believe that I'm withholding judgment.

"I don't know," he stares down at the carpet then up at me but I maintain the brick wall I've been building ever since my glass house shattered into brittle pieces. The wall that my mom said I should've always had up but never did, until now. Michael wants me to cry and plead with him to stay like I did the other times, but this time I can't. "I am going to visit her in Minnesota."

"I think that's a good idea." *In fact, this is his most rational idea yet.* "You should see what it's like before you rush into anything."

"You knew this was going to happen." His eyes are full of fake sorrow. "Well, I don't know what to do. I love her."

I listen, holding back my inner cry, refusing to give him the satisfaction. I'm starting to feel weak again. I want to give in. I don't want this divorce. I just want things to be back the way they were, but how can they be? The trust is gone, forever.

"Do you want to come live in Minnesota too?"

"What?!" I *did not* expect *this*. Does he want "Big Love" or something?

"They have better health care."

I'm wide awake now. "I never thought about that?"

"It's a chance for better health care for Bodhi," he nods off to the side.

"Maybe this is all for a reason," I say out loud. "To get Bodhi better healthcare? But I can't do anything right now because the kids' schools are working out so well for them."

"I know...I know," Michael solidly agrees.

After he leaves, I'm in alone in bed thinking. There are positives to this move. We'd all be together and even have real extended family close by. Then there is the Mayo Clinic. From what I've heard, it's more progressive when it comes to mental health care. Canada isn't far away. Healthcare is free if we move there. No longer would I have to worry about the costs of Jani and Bodhi's care. No water issue either. Here, we're in a drought.

And in a way, it's kind of exciting. I would be a lot closer to my good friends Marilyn, in Missouri, and Bethanne back east. Also, I'd like to meet all these women like me who are working to change the laws for the mentally ill. They gather in Baltimore and D.C. It would be a lot easier to do all of this from Minnesota.

CHAPTER 41

NO ROOM FOR DADDY

September 2015

Marty had to leave. He's one of Bodhi's favorite behaviorists, but he's off now, leaving me alone with Bodhi and Friday. We're waiting in the parking lot by the Guitar Center while Jani takes her singing lessons. I really need to save money and it would be easier if we didn't have to make this drive. Bodhi, like Jani, HATES waiting in the car and Friday comes with me everywhere these days because, believe it or not, he has separation anxiety too.

The lessons are only about 25 minutes, but that's enough time for Bodhi to go crazy on me. He's already fidgeting around so I give him his Geodon and Benadryl. Thank God he takes it. Then I bring up his crayons, paper, cars, trains and carry-on tracks, but even those are not enough. He's restless again. "I wanna go!"

God, he sounds like Jani. I put on some music. "Do you want to go to Del Taco?"

"No."

"Are you sure? Not even for a strawberry shake?"

"There's no room for Daddy," he blurts out. This, I did not expect to hear.

He looks around the car, then up at me with pleading blue eyes, like he's trying to make sense out of Daddy not being around as much as he used to. He's incredibly lucid, looking over at Friday occupying the seat next to him. I have the cup holder down, dividing the backseat in two but Bodhi knows that all I would have to do is lift it up, tucking it back into the seat, and there would be room.

"Daddy's in Lancaster." I know he needs more. He's ready to hear it. "Bodhi," I say, seriously. "You know Mia, right?" I look into his eyes and I've got him. He nods. "Daddy fell in love with her and he is making a choice to be in Lancaster right now."

"I want Daddy!" he cries.

"I know you do but I want you to know that this isn't your fault, or Jani's fault, or my fault. This is just the choice Daddy is making because he fell in love with Mia. But he is coming to visit you tomorrow." Bodhi looks at me, completely present in this moment, slowly scrunching up his face, his lower lip pouting out. Then comes the loud, painful cry. I leave my seat and move to the back with him, holding him close to me. He's always been so easy to love. No one ever talked to me about this part, when special needs kids go through a divorce. This is so hard to go through. Sometimes, I want to give up but it would all be worse for Jani and Bodhi if I were gone too. I'm forced to go through this painful mess with them.

"I want a strawberry shake," Bodhi says, decisively. Just like Jani, he changes the subject on me when it gets too deep. The truth is there is nothing left to say.

*   *   *

The next day Michael comes over, clearly distracted, but he still takes the kids on their usual dinner adventure to Wendy's, brings them back, then leaves. He doesn't say "Goodnight" this time.

At least I don't have to deal with his moods anymore. He's always in some sort of "crisis" and it's nerve-wracking. It's actually more peaceful after he leaves now. It's weird because I used to always feel safe when he was with us and now I feel nervous, like I don't know what's going to happen next, and there's ALWAYS something coming next. Not even an hour goes by before he calls from his drive back to Lancaster, crying. "Please divorce me now! Mia's threatening to break it off if I don't move to Minnesota."

He can't shock me anymore because I always expect some sort of drama from him and it's always overblown. "Here's what we can do," I tell him, "We can get divorced but you need to stay in California for at least a year or two so Bodhi has more time to stabilize on the right medication and Jani is in high school. She just started 8th grade. You'd be putting too much stress on both of them."

"You're right," he sniffles. At this point, I feel more like his mother than his wife. I post this new resolution on Facebook.

"Michael and I were talking and we've decided that we're going to give Bodhi a year or two to stabilize before he and Mia begin their 'Happily Ever After' life in Minnesota." I can't help sounding bitter.

*　　*　　*

"I hope you're happy now!" I wake up the next morning to an angry voicemail. Apparently, Michael hadn't told Mia about our solution and she read it on my page. Now she's giving him a more urgent ultimatum. If he doesn't move by June, she's breaking it off.

"So much for your 'true love.'"

"You know, I really despise you."

"Look, I have to deal with Bodhi asking where you are almost every morning. He was so used to stumbling all over you in the living room and now there's just an empty space. Do you realize how many times I hear 'where's Daddy?' All I can say is, 'Daddy's in Lancaster.'"

His anger turns adolescent. "If I lose my relationship with Mia, I will never forgive you!"

"I'm not IN your relationship with Mia. You two need to work it out. I'm staying here with the kids. And I've already decided there's no *way* I'm moving to Minnesota! The kids are too stable here. They have their behaviorists who are more than an extended family. Plus, the schools are excellent and they're basically happy."

I look at the progress both Jani and Bodhi have made during the time Michael's been in Lancaster. It's huge! Bodhi is talking more now. He's about three years behind his peers but he finally got that language explosion. Jani is also three years behind her peers. Not when it comes to speech but other skills, like conversational talking with her friends. In this way, they're both autistic-like, conversing much better with adults than kids their own age.

CHAPTER 42

TAKE MY EYES OUT

October 2015

"I'm afraid of the dark!" Jani runs into our room, panicking. She can't sleep. Now she sounds like Bodhi, who is also restless in his little bed. At least there's a rational explanation for all of this: Michael. He hasn't been around or even called for two days.

I feel God's presence filling me with the strength and energy I need to get through this moment and be strong for my children. "Do you want to sleep in here with us?"

"No." Jani's voice is trembling. "Can you sleep with me?"

"I can, but you'll have to wait until Bodhi is completely down for the night." I get up and give Bodhi his Benadryl, Jani her Thorazine, and take another Klonopin for me. Now all three of us are sandwiched in bed together. I let my body drive me through the motions.

Bodhi's light snoring is our cue. I gesture Jani back into her bedroom where I lead her through the deep breathing exercises we learned from Michi back when she was four. A few hours later, I wake up with my "Ball of Bode" snuggled up next to me. The three of us are sandwiched together again, this time sleeping on Jani's bed.

How in the world am I going to balance two special needs kids, with different needs at different times, *by myself*?

*   *   *

I dread Wednesdays.

"I have my singing lessons," Jani dances out of her room.

"I don't wanna go," Bodhi wails.

"I'll NEVER get to my singing lessons!" Jani screams.

I'm stuck. I've already canceled so many of Jani's lessons and they're not cheap. "Okay," I say firmly. "We're going." I grab Bodhi's hand and walk straight forward with Jani by our side. I really didn't want Friday to come too but he slipped through the door while I was distracted and I don't have time to put him back.

The forty-five-minute gap between behaviorists is just killing me but I have to do this because of their rules. They can't drive in the car with us. They have to meet us at the location but it doesn't make sense for me to have them come because it's too short of a time. They are supposed to allow 15 minutes to get to each place we meet. By the time they arrive at the Guitar Center, they have to leave. My new reality: Sometimes I have to go it alone. We're close to home, but Bodhi is ramping up, even after his Geodon and Benadryl.

I drop Jani off at the Guitar Center, then spin over to Del Taco, hoping he'll eat 500 calories to make the Geodon works. "Can I take your order?" The lady in the voice-box speaks to me while Bodhi squirms out of his seatbelt.

I'm calm in the middle of the storm.

Friday doesn't seem to mind that Bodhi quickly escalated to raging around him. Honey wouldn't have either. There's something inherently understanding inside these shepherds that keeps *them* calm in the middle of the storm even when I'm about to let *Jesus Take the Wheel* here, or at least Carrie Underwood.

Why am I here? How did it all come to this? I CAN'T DO

THIS ANYMORE!

"Uh, yes," I say, to the voice-box lady as Bodhi tumbles around. Now I feel him behind me on the floor of the backseat. That's a good place for him. He's safer there so I just call back to him like any other parent would do. "Bodhi, do you want a cheese quesadilla or a bean and cheese burrito?"

"Burrito," he answers from the middle of his own, personal Fight Club. I know this is not his fault.

Then, I wait for the lady to ask what else we want. This is taking too long. "Bodhi, sit in your seat, NOW! Do you want red or green sauce?"

"Green."

"Green," I repeat to her.

As I pull up to the window, the lady is sympathetic, having seen my plight in the car while we were waiting for other customers to be handed their food. She's a young girl, newer to the world than me in so many ways, yet she seems to understand.

"He's so cute," she compliments Bodhi.

"Thank you. I believe he's schizophrenic and not on the right medication," I just blurt out to her, letting my tears fall freely.

"I have a friend who's schizophrenic and she *has* to be on her meds."

"I know." She is compassionate. When she takes my hand in hers, I roll down the window for her to see Bodhi. "Bodhi, say hi." Usually, he will do this, but this time he doesn't. I nod off to the side as she hands me the bag of food.

"It's okay," she smiles.

I start to drive off...then come to an abrupt stop, noticing that Bodhi is halfway out the window! "SHIT!" I get out of the car and force him back in, then quickly roll up the window and put the child-safety lock back on. I have no one to blame but myself, so I stare into the video camera above me and scream. "This is NOT autism! This is PSYCHOSIS!"

"You'll be okay, sweetheart," the kind lady says, waving good-bye. "Take care." Those small gestures settle me down. I wish I could stay calm in the middle of all the storms but they just keep coming at me. I pray for a rainbow.

*   *   *

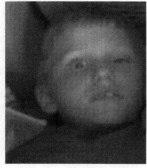

"I want to scratch my eyes out," Bodhi says, eating his food. He's settled down as we wait for Jani. He says this a lot. Usually, it's just "Take my eyes out," so I guess I should be happy that he's using more language. "I wanna go to UCLA." He's crying. He knows he can't control it and I'm only making it worse by how I'm reacting, but I'm past my breaking point. So, I break the behaviorists' rule of ignoring that request. I'm in survival mode and he is always at peace when we are on our way to UCLA, just like Jani used to be. "Okay, we'll go back to UCLA but only if you're good," I play along.

Bodhi right after we got home from Jani's lesson.

He gets back into his seat. "I'm good." The idea of going back to UCLA automatically comforts him and will get us back home safely. I breathe a huge sigh of relief when I see Jani fly out the Guitar Center doors.

*   *   *

When I get home, I notice that Stanford called. I have been trying to reach them for months now. All I want is for Bodhi to get an inpatient Clozaril trial to see if it works. If it doesn't, then I'll leave everything alone. There is a four-month waiting period and all they need is a referral from Dr. Maki to begin the intake process. The plan is to try the Clozaril there but have it monitored outpatient by Dr. Maki in Los Angeles. If only that were to happen.

Chapter 43

Cold Feet

Halloween 2015

"You've never missed Halloween with the kids," I remind Michael. I'm scared he's actually going to leave me alone with both of them this Halloween night because Mia is back in California. I guess Michael wasn't moving fast enough, so she came back. "You can always come too, Mia." My offer is serious. It's much easier when she is with us because of the three-to-two logistics.

Michael looks at her, waiting for permission. "I'm going to miss Lia trick-or-treating too."

"But it's a Saturday night. Do you guys have any plans yet?" Michael shakes his head. Mia shrugs "maybe" and we leave it at that.

*   *   *

There's a sad chill in the air this Halloween night. We're trick-or-treating in the same neighborhood with our support group friends who are our family. Jani wants me to dress up as the Queen in *Brave* so I used an old emerald-green maid-of-honor dress from my friend Marilyn's wedding. I accent it with gold costume jewelry and do my best to masquerade fun.

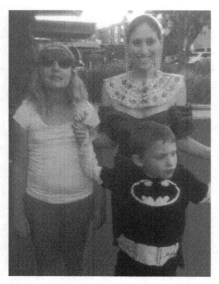

The Schofield Three ready for trick or treating.

When it's dark enough to go out, Bodhi gets scared. Here he is, the cutest little Batman, passed out on the couch of Ian's mom's home. I would stay here with him but he wakes up as soon as everyone is ready to go out and tells me he wants to sit in the car. Jani has never been scared. On the contrary, she's excited. If only Michael and Mia were here instead of making a "statement" that they're a couple and come first in each other's lives.

As we head to the door, my hand is tightly wrapped around Bodhi as he squirms to get away. Ian's Mom stops us to hand Bodhi a bag full of candy. "I want to go to the car," Bodhi gives a warning cry, making me look up at Jani. She demands to go trick-or-treating.

I stand in one place while I think this through but Ian's mom is way ahead of me. "I can take Jani," she offers. "You go with Bodhi. He'll probably eat the candy in the car."

"Thank you," My masquerade of fun is wearing thin.

"No problem. I get it." And she does. So few people understand this dilemma. If I DO take Bodhi around the block, he will be screaming, terrified, falling down on the cement. I am guaranteed another CPS visit. If I DON'T take Jani then *she* will be out-of-control, thrashing on the ground, screaming. That would also bring another CPS visit or, worse, a police officer because of her age. All this makes me hate Michael even more than I already do but I can't think about that now. Instead, Bodhi is loaded up with candy and we sit in the car listening to music while Ian's Mom takes Jani trick-or-treating. Anyone who can handle Ian can definitely handle Jani.

*   *   *

Jani called me three times from school today, wanting to go home early. I can only assume it's related to our pending divorce. Later she tells me, "I don't mind you getting divorced. I mind that Daddy's moving to Minnesota."

"I feel the same way." Jani and I are bonding on a whole new level now. Neither one of us can really speak, but we feel each other's pain by osmosis. "At least it's peaceful here now." Too bad it doesn't last. Barely an hour later, Michael bursts through the door like he's running away from a storm blast.

"Where's Mia?" I ask.

"She doesn't know I'm here," his breath is heavy. "I miss my family! I just got a note from Jani's teacher and wanted to make sure everything was okay." I asked her teacher to send Michael a progress report because they were just coming to me.

He's as sweet as a sugar, hugging Jani. Then he goes over to Bodhi, who we think is sleeping but he comes awake like he's been expecting Daddy any minute. We all take Friday for a walk. It's a beautiful night. *Is this a sign that he's coming back to us?* It all comes down to next week. Will he go or will he stay? Michael has never stayed a full booked ticket as long as I've known him. He's set to leave Wednesday, November 11th and return Tuesday the 17th. If I'm right, he'll be back by Sunday, Monday at the latest, but if I'm wrong then I truly have no idea where this is going.

I finally stop Jani's singing lessons, promising her we will get a second dog as soon as Michael moves. I just can't put myself or Bodhi through another one of those sessions.

*   *   *

On Wednesday, Michael is set to leave for the airport but makes another surprise visit instead. He stops short in the living room where we all gather around. He looks at me like he's near death. "My white blood cell count is high."

The Old Me would start fearing the worst and try to comfort

him but I hold back from running over and wrapping my arms around him. The New Me is hesitant in every move I make. He wants me to cry for him. *I want to cry for him.* I just refuse to do it anymore. It would be a repeat of the Scarlet situation and I'm too tired to go through another drama. Instead, I ask "How high is it?"

"Seventeen."

"You know there's leukemia in your family." *It's clear that's what he fears.* "Wait a minute. That's what Jani's was when we were going to move back in together, remember? Stress related anxiety. Clearly, you're under a lot of stress right now." I don't mention it's self-inflicted. Not that it matters anyway, he's still intent on making this trip to Minnesota to see the "love of his life."

*　　*　　*

Jani's new obsession is looking up the weather in Minnesota. We're icy cold here and it's just dipping into the 40s. Minnesota has been dropping below zero, but she tells me today is in the 30s.

"Just think, Jani, you would hardly ever be able to wear short sleeves or skirts. And you hate jackets and even long pants." She's a lot like me. The less clothes, the better: a California girl through and through. There's another problem with moving to Minnesota: I *cannot* drive in the rain. How would I ever be able to drive in the snow? We really are all better off staying here.

"Daddy's calling from Minnesota!" Jani happily holds up her pink iPhone.

"What's he doing?" I ask, my curiosity getting the better of me.

"He wants me to talk to Lia. They're at a park," Jani tells me, trying to talk to four-year-old Lia. There's not much back and forth between them. I listen and laugh-cry. Shouldn't he be at a park with Jani and Bodhi? I can't seem to get past Michael doing all of this but with each passing day, the fantasy Michael and Mia created becomes more of my reality. I guess he never really loved me the way I thought he did.

*　　*　　*

Michael returns on the 17th as planned. He had a good time. So much so that when Jani and Bodhi start fighting, he says how much he misses Minnesota already. He's already booked his next flight!

"What about Bodhi's birthday party?"

"I won't be able to make it. I had to go with the cheapest tickets, but I'll still be home for his actual birthday." I bite my lower lip. The old Michael would never put his kids second, but I guess that Michael is gone now. Or maybe he never existed at all.

CHAPTER 44

LIFE SUPPORT

November 2015

I would not be able to survive Michael's whirlwind metamorphosis without my behaviorists. They're not just ABA therapists, but lifelong friends and, more importantly, an extended family. At times they're breathing for me, letting me rest during their time with Bodhi because they know he's up most nights, leaving me little chance to sleep.

Jani's still watching movies and I make sure to get her a new one every time I'm at the store. Whenever I stop to think, I wish I hadn't. The pain is too great. It's overwhelming, and there's no time to cry. How can I break down if I'm the only constant in my two children's lives?

*   *   *

"I told Jani that I'm moving to Minnesota," Michael says, pity washing over his blue eyes.

"Why do you keep telling her this? She knows that."

"Yeah, but I don't think she really believes it." *God, he's like a bee that won't stop stinging.*

"I'm just curious. What will you do if you have leukemia?"

"I'm not changing my plans."

Brave man. "What about health insurance?"

"That's why I'll have to get a job with health insurance in Minnesota because my insurance here won't work there." Can't argue that logic.

"Well, that's just what you have to deal with, I guess. Anyway, we're looking at getting another dog when you move. Friday needs a brother or sister. He won't let me go anywhere in the car alone. And it will help distract Jani."

"Are you sure you can afford that?"

"No, but I don't know what else to do at this point. So, when are you leaving?" I redirect the conversation.

"I'm hoping to leave in January, after Jani's IEP." A wave of rough water rushes through me. This is all happening so fast. My body is no longer my own. The water is taking me wherever it wants me to go. I knew this tidal wave was coming but I didn't know how intense it would be to ride through it.

*   *   *

"Is everyone ready to go to Wendy's?" Michael asks Bodhi, with Mia by his side.

"I want ALL of us to go," Bodhi states. A perfect sentence!

"You mean, Daddy, Jani, and Mia?" Michael clarifies to Bodhi swinging on the edge of his spinning chair.

"No. Mommy too," Bodhi reiterates like Michael didn't hear him the first time. This is killing me. I want so much for Bodhi to understand everything, to be as neuro-typical as possible, but when he is, it's heartbreaking. He's so perceptive of the new dynamics.

Michael and Mia look over at me but I can't say much because I actually want them to take him and give me a break. But *he* won't go if *I* don't go and then *Jani* will be upset because she won't be able to go and then Michael will yell at Jani and everything will just go to Hell. So, I tag along for the ride, letting Mia sit in the front while I sit in the back with the two kids. It's just easier this way.

* * *

The next morning, we listen to the radio while I drive them to school. Jani attributes meaning to every song that plays. This is a good thing because it is age-appropriate and helps her process everything. As for Bodhi, I don't know what's really going on in his mind so I just take Melinda's advice. "I love you Bodhi," I tell him through the rearview mirror. "You're a good boy." Then I turn to Jani, next to me. "And Jani, you know you're a good girl and how much I love you." I look back at Bodhi again. He seems so well-adjusted in this moment. I'm just an ordinary single mom taking my two ordinary kids from their broken home to school.

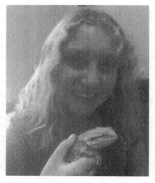

"I want you to know that Daddy leaving is not any of our faults. It's not my fault, it's not Bodhi's fault, it's not Jani's fault, or Friday's fault...."

"Or Ryder's fault, or Midnight's fault," Jani continues, ending with her hallucination cat.

"Daddy fell in love with Mia and she lives in Minnesota and he wants to live

Jani and Ryder in 2015. with her there."

"Mommy stays with us forever," Jani says.

"Yes," I turn to her and smile. "I'm your Mom and I will always be here for you. You're my kids. You both come first."

* * *

"Are you okay?" Michael turns to me before heading back to Lancaster. His movements are slow, solemn, subtle. Mia's waiting for him in the car. This is what she usually does now while Michael finishes reading to Jani.

"Look at me," I shake my head from side to side. "Do I look okay?" All I wear now are Target pajamas disguised as comfortable clothes. They're cheap, with built-in bra tank tops, so I can fall asleep at a moment's notice. That's really all I get.

He shrugs. "What are you *not* okay about?"

Is he just stupid? I was always told there are no dumb questions, but this *has to* break that rule. "Uh…the divorce…the kids being so affected by the divorce…." Michael nods. "Should I go on?" He looks pitiful, so I continue. "Friday not leaving the car. I have to take him everywhere and make sure the window is down. What am I going to do in the summer? I can keep all the windows down, even put water in the cup holders, but it gets over a hundred degrees outside! And he won't stay in the apartment alone."

"You know…if I could," his sweetness returns, "I would give you more money. If I was making four grand, I'd be happy to give you two grand."

His response is more money? Well, okay, I'll go with that. "But what about Mia? That wouldn't make her happy."

"No, she wouldn't be happy," he giggles sarcastically. This is all way too funny. "I'm serious. I would do that."

"So when are you leaving, permanently?"

"January 31st." Sadness seeps through my skin. It's weaker since he told me the twenty years he spent with me were miserably long and he felt like he was dying. With Mia, he feels free.

"So you really are planning to marry her?"

"Yes."

I'm desperately trying to finish this mourning process, but it's just not happening.

CHAPTER 45

A STOLEN LIFE

December 2015

"Read this! It describes Michael's relationship with you and the kids." Melinda sends me links to articles and books about "narcissistic" fathers. They keep popping up on my phone while we talk, but I'm used to it. I get this from my friends all the time now, especially the ones who didn't know Michael and me in the early years. *They don't see that he wasn't always like this!* "You were in Stockholm Syndrome with a narcissist."

"That's what Warrior Mom told me a long time ago, before she reported me to CPS." Warrior Mom never knew us in real life either, but Michael wrote blogs about our life and even though a lot of them were exaggerated, she thought he was a narcissist. "It's not like he's always been that way." My voice gets weak.

"There's more to it. Just read the article." Melinda is so insistent that I actually hear her gritting her teeth through the phone. She is right about so many things but sometimes she treats me like a child. I listen to her advice and we go over the questions together. She thinks they all apply to Michael, and most of them do to some degree NOW, but not as much in the earlier years. *Or maybe, it's just that I didn't notice?*

"You already told me he doesn't take criticism well and believes he's entitled to only the very best."

"That's true, but Michael doesn't 'set out' to hurt people." My defenses are up again. *This can't all be true?* "A lot of it's because of the life we've been living. That's when things started to fall apart and he started going into these rages. I made him get on Lexapro, which he did FOR ME!"

"Fine. Whatever." I hear Melinda's shallow sarcasm hanging over the phone line. It makes me think back to when he was adamant that he was "stuck in traffic," then his later admission that he really WAS with Scarlet while Jani waited for him. "Okay, looking back, I can see what you see. I was never as important to him as he was to me, but somehow I got used it. I never had a real relationship before so I never knew what 'normal' was supposed to be like. My feelings for him really changed after he broke his promise to Jani."

*   *   *

December 4th is a special day. It's the twentieth anniversary of our first meeting back in 1995. By the end of my KFI shift, Michael smiled at me as he walked into the editing bay and said, "You're cute." I returned the compliment and within days, we were dating. Now, twenty years later, our daughter is performing in the class choir. Her second mainstream class! Pam wants to see the concert too and helps Jani get ready for it. Now she sits in the middle of us, like a referee.

Bodhi's too unstable to be here but at least we have two respite workers who can watch him long enough for us to attend this event. Jani's been talking about it for months and is adamant about both us being here to see her perform. I'm glad we can because Michael's leaving next month for Minnesota and who knows what the future will bring. She's come so far even since she walked up on stage to receive her 6th-grade diploma. I can't believe all that happened in the last two years.

"You know," I look over at Michael, feeling sentimental, "It's exactly twenty years since the day we met." I smile with pride over at Jani. No matter what, look at what we've created. There was a time when we didn't know if Jani would make it out of the hospital, then to her special education classroom, and even further to the mild to moderate autistic class. Now, she's functioning in a mainstream class and doesn't look a bit out of place!"

But Michael just looks dully back at me. "You took twenty years of my life." I swallow hard, then look over at Pam, sinking into the seat between us. There were so many other responses I'd expected. Actually, I don't even know what I'd expected, but this didn't even enter my radar. I continue to watch Jani with pride. I got two beautiful children out of the last twenty years and I love them with all my heart and soul.

CHAPTER 46

YOU DON'T WANT ME ANYMORE

December 2015

Michael's on his second visit to Minnesota and Jani is having mini breakdowns. Like me, Jani is still grieving, but her grief is further fueled by teenage angst and hormonal changes. She has yet to become a woman but at nearly thirteen and a half, we're getting close.

Our kitchen is small and she's as big as any adult now so we constantly bump into each other. "Here, why don't you finish your cooking and then I'll come in and do mine." She loves cooking and *I love* that *she loves* cooking because I don't. I want *out* of the kitchen as soon as possible.

"Fine! You don't want me anymore!" She runs off, slamming the door.

"No, that's not true!" I twist the doorknob, but it's locked. I don't trust what she can do in this moment. "You *have to* open the door or I'm calling the paramedics!" She opens the door. Clearly, she's been crying. This is so neuro-typical, it makes me crumble. "Here, we'll both do the cooking. You stand by the refrigerator and give me a few minutes. I'll finish my part, then you take over. Okay?"

I so wish we had a house with a large kitchen. I never anticipated Jani loving to cook as much as she does. Eventually, I'll let her do it all. She is that good. In fact, next semester she's going into mainstream advanced cooking. When her teacher told our IEP team that some mainstream kids aren't ready to advance but she is, I beamed.

I know part of her behavior is my fault. I made a big mistake last time by telling Jani that Daddy always comes back from a trip early. When he didn't, I decided to handle it differently, telling her, "No matter what, he will always be your daddy and Bodhi's daddy. But, I do need you to know I can never take him back as a husband. Too much has happened and I cannot trust anything he says anymore and a relationship needs to be built on trust." I needed to make this clear for her and for me.

In the depths of these moments, Jani is completely present and well thought out. "No, you can't." I need her to understand this because she may get married at some point and I want her to know how important trust is in every relationship. Without it, there is no relationship.

Bodhi has fewer meltdowns but his disorganized thinking is getting worse. Thank God he's talking more and his communication is better all the time. Because of the psychosis, what he says doesn't always make sense. It's a never-ending battle to get him on the medicine that helps Jani walk through our world uninterrupted.

Michael is back in time for Bodhi's annual IEP meeting and it is reminiscent of three years ago. Aileen, his first school psychologist back in preschool, leads the team. "Bodhi recognized me right away," she says, warmly. "He ran up to me saying 'Miss Aileen!'" Everyone is there including Daria and all of his goals are being met. He still has a ways to go but he is definitely on an upward swing. The pride I feel is euphoric as I look over at Michael. I wish he shared my pride in our son, but even though he's sitting right next to me, it's like he's not here.

Later, I gauge Bodhi's thoughts about all of this. For him, I use more questions, mostly because I want to know what his thoughts are since he has so much trouble expressing them. "Daddy will always be your Daddy, wherever he is, Bodhi. You know that, right?"

"Yes."

"But if Daddy ever decided he wanted to come back to me as a husband, do you think should I take him back?"

Without a moment's hesitation, he says, "No."

I'm always amazed at how much Bodhi knows but keeps to himself. When I talk to him, if I am either the loudest or the most interesting voice, he comes back to center. The medication quiets the voices and dims the hallucinations so it's easier to focus and when he can focus, his communication is clear.

*   *   *

I am grateful for the incredible support team I have, especially when I'm sick. Most of the time I just move right through it but this time I can't even get up. Once again, my behaviorists are here and they save me until Michael comes back from his trip. It leaves me wondering how in the world I am going to make it without him. It doesn't take long before I gather the strength to know I can do it. He waltzes into my sick room, his hair disheveled and his shirt puke green, and starts negotiating child and spousal support.

"Look, I'm *sick*!" My voice cracks. "I'm just not up for discussing this right now." I get Melinda on the phone, my throat still scratchy. I can hardly speak. She hears this and now he's dealing with another Scorpio woman who becomes my voice. *Good Luck!* They go back and forth for a bit and both are getting frustrated.

"By the way, I didn't realize the court date was January 8th and the kids will be out of school. So, what are *you* going to do about that?" He says this as though they're just my kids and not his, but I'm way ahead of him.

"I've already scheduled respite for that day."

He offers a cold nod. "I can't pick them up tomorrow. I couldn't get anything done with them today."

"Huh?" It flies out of me. Welcome to my world! How could he forget how hard this is? Has he been gone that long? "You don't have to worry. All I needed was sleep. I know I'll be better tomorrow," I say, secretly worrying about the day I'm this sick again and he's not here. It's like he's pulling the plug on me. Somewhere along this journey, we both died. There was no funeral or memorial. We just re-emerged with altered souls.

CHAPTER 47

PASSION BY PROXY

December 2015

"Zach texted!" I tell Melinda over the phone "Just like he promised he would." I always forget how exciting this feeling is until it comes over me. Even if it's just for an hour or two, it gets my heart pumping, and now he's coming over. When I open the door for him, the same rush of adrenalin surges through me. Maybe Michael is right, maybe it is passion that keeps a relationship together, and I never had this kind of passion for Michael. "I have to go to the grocery store," I tell Zach, heading out the door with Alysha. "Bodhi needs snacks. You wanna come?"

"Sure," his carefree shoulders lift and I just want to fall into his arms and let him take over.

"Zach!" Bodhi's smile widens at the sight of the respite care worker who helped save him from himself during the worst times. Now we can share the best time. Michael's got Jani, so the timing is perfect to make our great escape but my phone soon interrupts my fantasy.

"Mommy, where are you?"

"I'm going to the store." I know she's with Michael so I'm careful what I say.

"What are you getting?" This girl is a natural reporter.

"Snacks for you and brother."

"I want rice for dinner."

"I can get that!"

"They only have the kind I like at Vons."

"Great, that's where I'm going anyway."

"Okay. Bye." Click. Jani's not one for long conversations.

*   *   *

A fresh-baked aroma wafts over us as we enter the bread section
at Vons. I've never it noticed before. "He's talking more," Zach says
as we pick out some vegetables.

"I know. Since you don't see him as often you really see how far
he's come, which is great." We're walking over to the snack aisle
with Bodhi when my mouth drops. *No! It can't be?!* I blink, blinded
by the blue dress shirt behind a shopping cart. *Why? Here? Now!*

"We needed to get rice!" Jani says, happily tagging alongside
Michael pushing the cart near the produce section. Michael knows
my attraction to Zach. He also knows that Zach is half my age and I
don't think it's a good idea for me to get involved with him, but
sometimes my hormones run away with me. I really don't know
what I would do if the opportunity presented itself.

"I'm getting the rice." I evil-eye Michael.

Jani smiles. She knows what she's doing. Can't I just have a little
"me" time to enjoy a feeling that I haven't had in years? "I can pay
for all of this," the "savior" says. Wow, Michael is being so gener-
ous? He must be reading my mind. "I just got a loan."

"For how much?"

"Three thousand. Jani told me you needed snacks so I've already
loaded up on them." I turn to Zach, who's a bit jumpy. I can practically feel what he's thinking: *What the hell am I getting myself into?
This is way over my head.* At the checkout line, Jani tells Zach she

wants him to ride back with her and Michael.

"No!" I say, a little too eager. "Zach's coming with me and Bodhi. Daddy just got back from being in Minnesota with Mia," I rush through my explanation. It's important that you have 'Daddy-Daughter' time."

Zach and I don't say much to each other on the ride back. He stays for a short time then hugs us all good-bye, until the next time. When that may be, nobody knows.

*   *   *

Our court date is looming in the distance and I was lucky enough to have Melinda convince me to talk to my mom about borrowing money for a special needs attorney. If I don't do this, Michael could run right over me.

"Do you want a cake pop?" I ask Bodhi while Jani and Alysha stand beside me. We're in front of the Starbucks inside Target. No answer. Usually, I follow up with "what kind of cake pop do you want?" but this time, there is no time. In an instant, Bodhi drops to the floor, arching his head back.

A second later, Aysha and I are down on the floor with him, in restraint mode. I hate dealing with this in public but it goes with the territory. I was thinking he needed to go back to UCLA anyway and I still haven't heard from Stanford, so I make the decision. "I'm taking him to UCLA." Alysha doesn't argue with me. She's in the middle of this too. She's on my side as I use my free hand to search for the liquid Benadryl in my purse. I need it to calm him down and as a cure if he goes into dystonia.

"Bodhi ran into the street yesterday," Jani bursts out from the sidelines.

"What?!" I turn to her, keeping a steady grip on Bodhi.

"Yesterday. Daddy lost him in the parking lot and cars were coming at him." Michael never tells me this stuff. Even Mia told me once when this happened in the mall parking lot. I'm getting angry that I can't even trust that he will tell me everything that goes on with the kids when I'm not around. I'm not asking for every detail, but this is important!

*   *   *

The day after Bodhi's admitted, Danielle calls with Karen, a new fellow who doesn't say much. I'm sure she's heard the rumors about us. Me, mostly. Michael doesn't get that angry in these sessions. He's the "easy one." It's *Mom* who's "the hard one." And, of course, it's the same story: no sleep, running up and down the halls, throwing poop, and laughing hysterically.

"You know," Karen says, "'Attention-Seeking' behavior." I hate this terminology because it diminishes psychosis. I mean, how many neuro-typical six and seven-year-olds are throwing their own poop, no matter how much they want attention?

"I think…" Michael starts out.

"What he's doing is CRAZY!!!" I interrupt, exhaling a deep breath.

"Can I get out a word in edgeways?"

"No!" I blast him.

"I think," he strengthens his voice, "that he has severe autism."

I turn to Michael. "He is getting all the ABA therapy that is possible. We are treating that!"

"Then it isn't working?"

"RIGHT. Because he's not autistic. He's schizophrenic! He can do well, just like Jani, with the ABA therapy, when he's in his RIGHT MIND!" Like I said, Michael's the easy one. Not me.

"Well, I don't agree."

I shake my head and wave him off. I know this irritates him but do I care? Nope. "Look," I talk directly to Danielle and the new fellow under Dr. Hyde, "I have the perfect idea to test your theory that it's 'Attention-Seeking Behavior.'"

"How?"

"By *ignoring it*! Then, you can see if it stops. You know, because he won't be receiving any 'attention' for 'the behavior. If it stops, then your theory holds water. If not, it's BOGUS!"

*   *   *

The kitchen sink is overwhelming me. So many dishes are piled up. It's a pet peeve of Michael's but that's not what I'm worried about right now. After a long morning in court, I'm actually pretty relaxed washing them. Bodhi is still inpatient but we managed to mediate it out, coming to a reasonable agreement that makes the judge happy too. Less work.

"Do you feel like you've won, today?" Michael asks, staring at me washing the dishes.

"What? We came to a settlement today."

"Well, I got hammered by Mia. She says that I'm being more loyal to you than her because I gave you spousal support."

"You wouldn't have done that if my parents didn't take $5,000.00 off of a credit card to hire an attorney."

"You know I don't have the money. How am I supposed to live?"

"Aren't you living with her parents? For free?!"

"We can't do that forever. Besides, they said they're going to charge me rent."

"Look, there are three of us and ONE of you. This is your obligation."

"My obligation is to the kids, not you!"

I throw my hands up in the air. "I'm disengaging." This is my new word when I'm tired of straining my voice in useless arguing.

"Well, I'm not going to be able to pay you," I hear him rattle off as I leave the room. *Didn't he just agree to this in court?*

*   *   *

A few days later, I get the call and I have no choice but to phone Michael. "Bodhi has an appointment at Stanford. It's scheduled for Friday, January 22nd."

"How are you going to get there?" Michael asks.

"I'm going to drive."

"By yourself?"

"Yes. Do I have any other choice? Would you and Mia like to come too?"

"No," he says, flatly.

*   *   *

That night I spot Dr. Hyde walking through the hallway so I approach him, more relaxed since I've gotten the appointment at Stanford now. "I know you're not going try the Clozaril, but can you at least retry Thorazine? He's been on the same medication for over a year now. I never thought he was allergic to it but at least now we can find out for sure."

"I can do that," he surprises me.

"By the way, I've got an appointment with Stanford for a Clozaril trial."

"Well, if they want to try it, then that's on them. But they can always call me." I don't know what to make of this, so I just nod, relieved that at least he's giving the go-ahead for retrying Thorazine.

The next day, the medication management nurse lets me know that they're going to give Bodhi Thorazine in the middle of the day to test it out. A few hours later, the call comes in that he *did not* have a negative reaction to it but instead had the best day he's had since he's been there. It works! I was right after all.

The two nurses were wrong. It *was* all because he was going off Risperdal at the same time. I knew this because, just like in the early years with Jani, I was skeptical about the medication, not knowing if he truly needed it. So, one morning I tried waiting longer than usual to give it to him but he went absolutely crazy and I had no choice. Once again, I learned that he's on medication for a reason: Because he really, truly has a mental illness and cannot survive without it.

CHAPTER 48

RE-HOMING

January 2016

"Where are you now, Daddy?" When I told Michael we were going to Stanford January 21st, he decided to leave for Minnesota the night before we left. That was nearly two weeks early.

"I'm in Nevada, Sweetie."

"It's cold." Jani already checked the temperature there. She's been calling Michael three times a day, maybe more. Her communication skills over the phone have greatly improved and she sees me role-modeling strength and determination, making this five and a half hour drive on my own. Those are both positives from this whole thing.

Meanwhile, I'm running out of gas and I have no money to spare. We left Friday in boarding because we don't know how long our short trip to Stanford will actually be. Ryder is relatively easy since he's just a one-year-old bearded dragon. Melinda said her kids would love to take care of him. We bought him a travel carrier and are dropping him off at her house.

"Is the gas light on?" Melinda asks over the cell, clearly annoyed.

"It's been on. I just don't know how low it can go."

"Well, how long has it been on?"

"About an hour, I think, but we've been stuck in traffic."

"Oh, God." Melinda's getting mad at me now. She's treating me like one of her children again and I'm older than her! "Where are you?! We live near the Six Flags that used to be Great America."

"I know. I know! I'm almost there." I remember going to Great America on so many field trips with my school friends. I was lucky enough to grow up with the same kids from kindergarten through high school. It wasn't always easy, but I do want this for Jani and Bodhi. "I see the Lawrence Expressway! I'm really close." Melinda gives me the exit and I'm happy to be on the road even though I'm chugging along on fumes at this point. "Okay, getting off," I say, exiting the turn off with the car coming to a slow crawl.

"Go to the nearest gas station and I will meet you there."

I know I'm on the last bit of gas as I glide into the Chevron station. "I'm here! I made it!" I'm so lucky that Melinda is here to meet me. I've always been low on money but even more so since Michael left. She gives me $40 for gas.

*   *   *

We enjoy a bit of sanity at Melinda's home with all her dogs and her normal life. It's weird, though, because I don't know if I could ever be this normal. I think there's a reason, well, I know there's a reason, I left for Los Angeles. It's because I'm crazy. I recognized right away in all the television shows I would watch as a child. These kid actors were like me. I'm not talking about the characters they played. I could see inside of that. I related to them as people and I wanted to be just like them.

That's why I didn't stay in San Mateo. It was just too boring. In our present, as Melinda walks the three of us out to my car, she tells me, "You know, sometimes boring is good."

"I know it is." I say the words she expects, but I remember telling my mom that if I ever had a regular job I would go crazy and kill myself. I really am bipolar. Melinda doesn't believe me, though. I guess when we were in high school I did a good job of hiding my real self. Michael wasn't the only one with daydreams of grandeur.

The flip side is that I don't have the security she has with her new husband. Now, I yearn for that too. My phone rings. "Who is it?" Melinda asks as I'm about to drive away from her home.

I tilt my phone toward her. "Scarlet again. I never blocked her. I guess somehow I feel guilty over all that happened."

"You should answer it."

"I want to, but I'm scared. It's been over a year and a half. It's not like I don't feel bad for her. I do."

"She probably just wants closure."

"I know," I sigh, my impulsiveness taking over. "Hello?" I hear her shallow breathing before the line goes dead. "She's been calling at least once a week, sometimes several times during the day and night. It's not just me but Michael too. And she's still under a restraining order."

"I wanna go!" Jani squeals while Bodhi pulls a blanket over his head to keep out whatever is disturbing him right now.

"We *are* going," I reassure her just as a text from Scarlet comes in. "I'm so sorry, pls forgive me." I text her back "I don't blame you. I blame Michael." I turn and tell Melinda, "I did it!"

"Good girl! You gave her closure."

*   *   *

On the drive to my mom's house, Scarlet's texts are coming in fast and furious. She's obsessed again. She wants my friendship back but after all that happened, I'm nowhere near any of that. If it was just her sleeping with Michael, that would be different. Eventually, I would be able to forgive her, but it's the "everything else." I can't trust her. I know she can't trust herself either. I really don't want to get back into this again so I call and ask Melinda what to do now.

"Just keep doing what you're doing. Remember, she was manipulated too. He wanted to re-home you."

"What?"

"You know, like a dog you find, but you can't or don't want to take care of? You try to re-home them." My heart has already been hurt by Michael, so really, what more could she tell me that would make it worse. "Remember, when you told me how Scarlet tried to set you up with her husband? How she and Michael both told you that her husband really liked you? Then, there was that mysterious fight between the three of them and her husband called you saying, 'I just want my wife back!'"

I think back to that strange call. "I thought it was because she was at our place all the time, helping out."

"They were always lovers…."

This hits hard. "What?"

"She would never have gotten this mad if it was just one time," Melinda states this as though it's fact. I'm in a new state of shock as I think back to all that led up to those moments with CPS, the police, and her accusing Michael of rape.

"You know, she also wanted to set me up with her father. She told me that he really liked me. I didn't know why she was pressing the issue because this was the last thing on my mind. Even Michael was urging me to talk to him. But Bodhi was in and out of trying to kill himself and Jani was just starting to stabilize."

"And then you liked Zach?" Melinda questions me.

"Well, yeah," I admit, on automatic rewind. "You know, one time when Zach was over playing with Bodhi, Michael said to him 'You can be my replacement.'"

"Weird."

"I know. But then," I still have to question Melinda here, because it's not like she knows everything about our life, "Why did Michael show up when I was with Zach at the store? Clearly, he was making a gesture that he wanted me back."

"Or he was just afraid to lose you. It's not the same thing. For twenty years, you've been each other's safety net."

*   *   *

The following morning, Melinda meets me at Stanford's Autism Clinic, not far from where she lives, so she can take Jani while my parents join me in the two-hour consultation.

The inside of the beautiful office is a miniature version of the autism clinic at UCLA. My parents settle in on the couch inside the kid-friendly office, complete with all the toy fixtures any child would want. We wait for the doctor to come out and meet Bodhi while he begins running up to different toys, then tossing them aside in favor of others. Nothing holds his interest.

"I wanna go now." Oh, how I remember this phrase before Jani was on medication. After I paid full price for her favorite play areas, she wanted to go in ten minutes. Nothing held her interest. This was the end of her beginning, before she was on medication. Finally, a pretty young Asian woman comes over to greet us and shake our hands before looking over at Bodhi.

"I get scared!" He covers his eyes, giggling. Then he removes his hands, squirming around on a little chair. "I get scared," he repeats, curling up into a ball. She smiles and shows us into her office while she talks to him alone.

"It shouldn't be long now," I tell my parents. "She's got to see what's going on here." She talks to him for a few minutes, then brings him into an office filled with more toys and a big train carpet mat. Bodhi plays quietly for a while.

"So, I have a questionnaire to go over." She smiles at me.

"Okay," I say, looking at my parents sitting off to the side. My mom is 75 and my Dad just turned 80. I'm so hoping this trip will be worth it but I'm tipped off early that this is not going to be what I thought it would. "So, you just met him. What do you think?"

"He's severely autistic," she smiles. "We see this all the time."

I sigh, hard and heavy. "Okay, let's cut to the chase here. I want a Clozaril trial for him. Is Clozaril tried on autistic children?"

"Sometimes…."

Bodhi begins throwing toys. He's bored again. We've been in

the consultation for ten minutes at the most. How we can get through two hours is beyond me, but at least she will see everything for herself. "Have you tried Prozac or maybe Risperdal?" she asks.

"Huh," I laugh. She just triggered me and I can't hold back. "Yes! We're waaaayyyyyy past Prozac and Risperdal. He was on that when he was four-years-old and it worked, for a while, then stopped working. Now, he is on 80 milligrams of Geodon, 600 milligrams of Lithium, and 75 milligrams of Benadryl daily. And it helps, but it's not enough! We just got Thorazine back, so that is helping too.

"Clozaril is a serious medication."

"I know it is. My daughter has been on it since she was almost 7 years old. She's 13 now and doing very well. She's also on Lithium and Thorazine."

In the middle of our conversation, Bodhi is getting out of control. "Maybe, your parents can take him for a walk."

I look over at my parents, every bit of their age. "There's no way they can take him for a walk now. Here, I'll give him a 25 mg of Thorazine and we can continue on." After going through part of the questions Bodhi has calmed down. "Did you notice how the Thorazine worked for him?"

"Yes, that's good."

"The problem is that it won't last that long. Two hours at best." She nods, sadly. "So, basically, all I would like to do is have him tried on Clozaril in an inpatient setting."

"Clozaril can have serious side effects," she shakes her head.

"I know that. This is why I want it done inpatient."

"He would have to go through the emergency room."

I'm crying inside. I look at my parents who have no idea what this means. "No, that's okay."

"Are you sure you don't want to do that, Susan?" My mom asks.

"I'll have to wait with both of them for at least six hours. Do you want to wait with me?" Both their jaws drop. My parents complain about a two-hour wait in the ER. They'll never be able to make this commitment. So, I decline, chalking it off to another failed attempt and maybe there is a reason that God knows and I don't. Maybe it wouldn't work on Bodhi. Maybe he would get the awful side-effects that Jani hasn't. I don't know anymore. All I do know is that I'm tired and at least Bodhi is on Thorazine.

*   *   *

It's pouring rain and Bodhi is sleepless again. I give him his meds, hoping that will do the trick, but it only lasts for so long. I don't know how much more of this I can take, especially, by myself. God, how I wish Michael was here, but he isn't. He just isn't.

I let Jani continue her peaceful sleep, just like when we're at home. There's so little space in the motel room that I have no choice but to take Bodhi out. Otherwise, it will be a nightmare. I hold his little hand, making sure I have the hotel key card tucked inside the pocket of my purse then leave the other one on the nightstand next to Jani, sleeping soundly thanks to the Clozaril. *Why does this all have to be so hard?*

*   *   *

Bodhi's footsteps slip over the splashy sidewalk and he laughs. At least he's having some fun in the middle of all this. I'm just grateful Melinda lent me her heavy coat to and thick Tamarac boots to wear. It's colder than I expected. Then again, it is 2 am.

The 24-hour IHOP is just a few feet away so we go there for an early breakfast. Maybe the Geodon I gave him will work, sending him back to sleep, if he'll only eat. But he won't.

I can't stop to think right now because I'll just cry and I'm not allowed to cry or be weak. Ever. If I stop, who will carry us on? I have to keep going here so I give my body the strength to take the next steps.

*   *   *

I find it ironic that I'm "cruising" the El Camino with my little boy. Thirty years ago, I was cruising with Melinda and my other high school friends for a very different reason. We were so young, looking for boys, no clue of what the future held for any of us.

297

Kaiser Hospital is up ahead. That's where I was born 46 years ago. I can see that it's been beautifully renovated even through the thick fog. I long to be home in Valencia, though. When it rains there, it's just rain and sometimes it's warm rain. I remember how much I dislike the fog but I now know this is going to be a short stay. It just reminds me how lucky I am. I may have challenges up the yin-yang, but I do love our home. It's spacious with majestic mountains just over the horizon and so many days of blue sky. It helps me, mentally, get through this.

As I continue driving, I think about how going home on Sunday will leave us no better off than when we came. It gets me angry. Why can't he just get a trial of the medication that's been helping Jani for years? There was a time when she didn't sleep but that all changed with the Clozaril.

*   *   *

I wasn't going to do this, but it just seems like a wasted visit if I don't. After being up all night, I call my Mom later that morning and tell her the news. We're already on our way to Stanford's ER. No one is coming with me. It's just too much to ask. Besides, I've been through worse and, right now, Bodhi is tired from being up all night so he's actually calm.

It's a smooth admission into the ER where they assure me that this will be the place we get the help we need. Only, we don't. Really, it's not their fault. While we're in the waiting room, Bodhi comes into the present. "I don't want to stay here!" He says, adamantly lucid as we're led into the ER room. And that's where we remain for 5 hours straight.

Bodhi is calmly restless while Jani is pounding on the door and kicking at it. And out she goes. I see her through the window, racing past the security guard. But I don't react. I'm too tired of reacting because that would just take energy away, leaving none left to spare. Jani is brought back to us by a nurse who shoves her into the room as Jani slams the door back at her.

A little while later, the psych doctor comes in and I'm getting ready to tell him how Bodhi needs to be on the same medication as Jani because…*it's helping her so much?* How do I say that now? Dr. Hyde really knew what he was doing when he let the medication management team retry the Thorazine. It works so well with the Geodon and Lithium. Basically, other than the sleep issue, Bodhi is stable. But Jani, a hormonal teenager who just lost her Dad to another woman half a continent away, is angry.

It's no surprise that there are no beds available. After our relatively short five-hour stay, I probably look the craziest with Jani coming in a close second. As for Bodhi, he's just fine. I sigh, looking up to God. I'm done asking for a Clozaril trial. This must be for a reason. Besides, I'm tired. I just want to go home, especially before they take Jani away.

Chapter 49

Renegades

February 22nd, 2016

On February 22nd, Scarlet writes me an eerie message. I'm at the dog park with Friday when I try to decipher what it means. "Today's going to be great! Wait, you'll see...for me too!" Later that morning I log onto my Facebook account and see her face planted on my page. She wants me to re-friend her again, so I comply with that part. I want to show her good faith, but what I really show her is how stupid I am.

Not an hour later, I try logging onto my Facebook again and I can't get in. It's down. They're telling me I violated community standards. I guess God has a reason for this, too? But I already know who's responsible and I don't have to look further than the Schofield Discussion page. This page grew out of an anti-psychiatry movement that began with Warrior Mom attacking us back in June 2009, after the first article about Jani was published in the Los Angeles Times. Scarlet was never anti-psychiatry but she took them whatever information she could and they ran with it. I'm not innocent in any of this and, sadly, I was even entertained for a while, but it's gone too far.

Sure enough, they proudly show off how they reported me for all the controversial stuff I've said, but it was probably posting screenshots of the Mia and Michael texts that got me into trouble. One had Mia's phone number. At this point, I'm done. I'm done with all of Michael's lovers and the haters he brought into our lives. They go around endless circles to keep their own minds occupied, which is, of course, all a part of mental illness. I get the hypocrisy on my part. But I've got two children to protect and Michael's gone. The kids are making progress, thriving even.

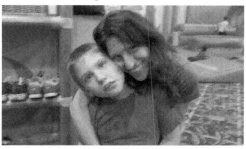

Susan and Bodhi at a birthday party for a friend of his.

I've also learned the power of choice. I'm choosing to no longer be a renegade. With this decision, I'm changing my phone number and buying a Tracfone. No more Mia with her antagonizing texts and no more Scarlet. My kids are too important to put at risk with all this nonsense. Besides, I want to be with the mothers, like Liza Long, whose article "I am Adam Lanza's Mother" went viral. Through all these years, I've finally learned how and why Columbine happened. It wasn't inattentive parents. Even the guns were secondary to the main issue. It was delusional thinking, mental illness gone untreated.

*   *   *

"How cold is it in Ithaca, New York?" Jani asks Siri on our drive to school. Jani's decided that she wants to know the temperature there since she's going to live with The X-Ambassador and that's where they live.

"Really," I laugh, thinking back to when I wanted to live with Duran Duran. I guess this is normal, maybe?

"I want to have five dads."

"Well, I wanted to marry John Taylor but the reality is that they are probably five guys who are in and out of their place and wouldn't have time for you. Not in the way you want, anyway."

"Yeah, but Daddy's a renegade." Michael arrived in Minnesota just after we returned home from the Bay Area.

"Jani, they say in their song that they're renegades."

"But Daddy's ruined my life." Neuro-typical, schizophrenic, autistic, it doesn't really make a difference. Divorce brings out the teenage drama queen (and manipulator) in any kid. Bodhi's in the back seat listening and I'm glad because he may not say anything, but at least he knows that all of us are in this together.

"It's not any of our faults. Michael fell in love with Mia and he wants to be with her in Minnesota. That's it." I know Bodhi feels angry hearing us talk and my heart sinks for him. He's only eight so he never got to know Michael as Dad like Jani did. I'm just grateful Michael left when he did versus a year or two before or, even worse, back in 2008 when Bodhi was just a baby. Then Bodhi would barely know him at all. But all of this comes with its own set of problems.

*　　*　　*

"Bodhi! Bodhi!! Mommy!!! Daddy's in California!" Jani's been chewing her pink iPhone charger so much the silver cord underneath is ripping.

It's weird how little effect Michael coming back is having on me this time. I'm not glad, mad, or even sad. I'm just like "here's Dad." Bodhi isn't faring as well. He's starting the downward slope I've become all too familiar with. He'll welcome Michael at first, then he'll retreat back, refusing to get into Michael's rental car, forcing Michael to take Jani alone before the three of them can go out together. This continues into Sunday. I don't know exactly when Bodhi started doing this but it is his "new normal." On Monday, Michael is about to leave again when Bodhi blasts into full, guttural tears. I'm lucky Alysha is here with me as we try to soothe him.

"I eat chocolate to cope," Jani says, pouring herself a bowl of chocolate cereal. She's gained so much weight since Michael's been gone. This is *not* the medicine.

"That's not good, Jani. It's actually good to cry," Michael urges her. He's not wrong but it is a quick fix, so I encourage it.

"Wait a minute!" I look over at Alysha who doesn't seem to be able to calm Bodhi either and Michael is just letting this go on and on. "I have an idea!" I say, loud and proud, "when Daddy leaves, we go get ice cream."

All of a sudden, Bodhi's eyes meet mine and Jani's too. "Yeah!"

"No," Michael protests. "They need to deal with their feelings."

"And they just did," I tell him, cheerfully. "Come on, kids. Let's go get some ice cream!" My kids follow me out, Alysha taking Bodhi by the hand, leaving Michael alone in the apartment.

*　　　*　　　*

"When Daddy leaves, we get ice cream," Bodhi sing-songs, through happy tears and strawberry ice cream at Ben & Jerry's. Jani joins in and now they're both singing. It's hard to shake the sadness of it all, but I have to. I don't have a choice in the matter. I have to model strength for them. At least I'm getting through the grieving process, but for Jani and Bodhi, it will never be over. He will always be their father.

Jani still hopes that Michael will return to being the father she once knew. The father I once knew and the father Bodhi never got a chance to know. Michael's not a "bad" person. I don't even believe in "bad people." He's given us good moments and I will never take that away from him. We could never have gotten here without him.

CHAPTER 50

GAME CHANGER

October 1st, 2016

A mutual Facebook friend sends me a new photo from Mia's page. I've managed to do what Bethanne told me a while back and blocked both of them for my own sanity. It's October 1st, but the photo was taken September 24th. It's Mia wearing an engagement ring from Michael. I can't say it's not another punch in the gut because I would be lying if I did. It hurts, every piece of it.

"I don't know why I didn't think of this before?" Melinda starts out. "I have this friend I've known for over twenty years. You two are so much alike." I listen with closed ears. "I want you to meet him. He's from Seattle."

"Melinda," I stop her with my hand up to the air. "You know I'm *not* moving from Valencia.

"I know that! He's willing to relocate. He just lost his job."

I give her a heavy sigh. "I don't have time for this."

"I wouldn't even bring it up if I didn't feel so strongly about you two meeting."

"Well, sure," I offer up my sarcasm, "if you two want to come down to help me out, fine."

"No, not me. I have four kids. I'm talking about Cory."

I laugh. "I'm not going to just meet some stranger! If you want me to meet him then *you* have to come with him!"

"Ugh. I have four kids," she repeats."

"Well, I have all the time in the world here," I shake my head, still frustrated that she still can't seem to grasp all that I go through in just one day, or even one hour. "Look, *you* pick the date and I will go with it."

"Okay." Wow, she's really serious about this. "He's coming to visit us this weekend since Nate has a meeting out of town. How about Friday?"

"Sure, perfect," I say.

*   *   *

Michael wants to modify the child and spousal support he promised to pay back in January, mostly the spousal support, so I've got yet another court date looming over my head. I'm in the middle of writing my letter to the judge when Melinda brings Cory into Fed-Ex. She's pissed off because I was supposed to be at my apartment. I guess I lost track of time. When she called from the airport, I really didn't think they'd be here so quickly. Usually driving from LAX to anywhere on the 405 takes forever.

"You said you would be at your apartment to meet us."

"Look, I have to get this letter done."

"I just spent $500.00 on coming here! I'm missing my kids' soccer games and swim team."

"I know you did."

"And you don't even appreciate it!"

"I do!" *God, I just wish she got my life.* I see Cory calmly standing in the background. I feel his energy. It's so calm, especially opposed to Melinda's right now.

"I'm leaving!" she dashes off.

"I do appreciate it!" I call out to her, then go back to the letter

I'm writing the judge. Cory stands behind me, unfazed by Melinda's reaction. "Can you read this over for me?" I finally turn to take a better look at him. He's tall and so normally nice looking. A breath of fresh air.

"Sure." He leans over me at the computer and reads my letter, closely editing some things I'd missed along the way. I'm so relieved. Meanwhile, Melinda is nowhere to be found but I know she just needs time to cool off.

When I'm done, Cory and I leave. He follows me back to my apartment in his rental car. We take Friday out to the dog park and our conversation is easy, as if we've known each other for years. About twenty minutes later, Cory texts Melinda and goes to pick her up while I wait with Friday at the dog park. After Melinda and I meet, we make up and go to Target where she shops for me. I must say, I'm a bit surprised by how easy everything is with the three of us. We go back to my place where Cory and I talk as Melinda puts away all the food and utensils she bought me.

What a great friend I have in her. We've known each other for thirty years now. She met Cory while we were in our twenties and out of touch. Melinda was working at the Emporium in Cupertino and Cory had just gotten a divorce from his wife who was in the Air Force. She was stationed in San Jose while they were raising their young daughter, Kelli. In fact, Melinda and Cory had been friends so long that he was the one who encouraged her to date Nate, now her husband of eight years.

Next is the real test: We drive to Jani's school to pick her up. All I've told her is that we're meeting Melinda and her friend Cory. After that, the four of us go to the Olive Garden. Since Bodhi's in the hospital, we can have a relaxed lunch, for the most part. We're even able to order drinks with regular glasses. But then..."I'm cold!"

"You want my jacket?" Cory offers, unfazed.

"No." Jani is whining. "I have diarrhea!"

"You can go to the bathroom, Jani," Melinda suggests.

"No, I can't. I need an Imodium."

"No, you don't. I just got you off of that. Now you have to continue. Your stomach looks great."

"I'm not sick?" Jani tells herself.

"No, you're not sick," I repeat back to her. The food comes and Jani eats along with the rest of us. I find out Cory's favorite food is Italian, just like mine. After dinner, Melinda and Cory have to rush back to the airport. When Jani and I are driving back home I ask her. "So, how did you like Cory?"

"I liked him," she smiles, adding an excited hand-clap, and I smile back at her. I never underestimate Jani. She knows exactly what's happening here.

*   *   *

A little later that night, while Jani's watching YouTube, I start to feel...something. Beyond Bodhi not being here, something else is missing. I think about the short time Cory and I spent together and how he handled Jani's screaming out about how she was cold and the feeling of diarrhea she had at the Olive Garden. It was a good sign, but a small sip of the full drink.

I know what I'm about to do is an impulsive move, but I don't hold back. And I don't know why I'm *not* holding back. This is *not* how I operate, but it's not my choice anymore. I'm hydroplaning on watery ground, holding on to the steering wheel not knowing when or where I will land, or if I will even come out alive. Tears well up over my head. I'm drowning.

I call Melinda in a panic. "Can you send Cory back?"

"I have four kids! I can't come back again." She misunderstands what I want.

"No, that's not what I'm asking."

She's still going on about how she has four kids, so I wait until she finishes, then slowly say, "That is not what I'm asking. I take a deep inner breath. "What I'm asking...is...if you can send Cory back *alone!*"

"Ohhh." *She gets it!* She doesn't seem as shocked as I thought she'd be. "Yeah, I can do that, but you have to give me some time.

We'll have to check the cheapest way to do it."

"I know." *Again, what the hell am I doing?* "Bodhi's not here," I tell her, "So Cory can sleep in Bodhi's bed next to mine. We're still going to take things slow, but I do like him."

"Okay, but you'll have to wait until tomorrow unless you want to pick him up at midnight."

Jani comes out of her room. "I want to read!"

This is our new nighttime routine. It used to be Michael's, but he's gone now and I have taken over where he left off. The only part I've changed is that we also read a passage from the Bible every night. I have never read it so we're still in The Old Testament.

"Okay," I tell Jani, then I'm back on the phone to Melinda, Jani standing by my side. "I'm trying to get Cory back. Would you like that?"

"Yes," she says, definitively, smiling. "I like Cory."

"Alright," I say, relying on my now fourteen-year-old daughter for the ultimate approval. If Jani disapproves, I cannot take this further. I vowed never to make Jani and Bodhi's life harder than it already is. "It will have to be the next bus out. Jani and I can't go tonight but we can get up early." I turn to Jani, "Is that okay with you?"

"Yes."

"There's one that leaves at 11 pm," Cory is now on the phone with me. "Can you pick me up at the Megabus in Burbank at 5:30 tomorrow morning?"

I turn to Jani, who's listening intently. "Is 5:30 am okay with you?"

"Yes," she says.

"Okay," I say, still unsure of what I'm doing. "Just call us as soon as you get there."

"I will."

"Oh, and just so you know, I'm going to get my Facebook page rocking again. I've been unusually quiet on there so I'm going to post something to keep it going. It's my personal therapy. My own little talk show. Then I'm going to read to Jani and go to sleep."

I can hear Cory grinning over the phone. "You know, I've seen it. I've just never responded."

I giggle like a fourteen-year-old. He seems to bring out this side of me, and that makes me feel happy. It's cool that he's actually six years older than me. To Cory, I'm a woman, not a mother figure like I was to Michael. "Ok, see you soon, sleep well," he says, sounding just as giddy as I feel.

*   *   *

"It's time for 'Facebook Datebook.' I know it's been a long time and, as usual, I'm going to sleep soon, but I'm just curious, is it a turnoff if your partner walks around naked?" Before I can even close my computer, Cory texts me. "I'm reading it now."

"LOL," I respond. This is kind of cool. It's like I'm actually on a date for the first time. I check my Facebook and I'm happy he is one of the men who does approve of a woman walking around naked. I know it's not for everybody but it is something I do sometimes, so I need any man I'm with to be okay with it.

Sunday morning, Jani and I get up at the crack of dawn to pick up Cory. He's waiting anxiously, stepping on and off the curb. There's no missing him. I let Jani choose where Cory sits in the car. She's as excited as I am but her feelings come first. "I'll sit in the back," she says.

Cory talks to us all the way home, mostly about the Seattle Seahawks, and Jani loves it. He distracts her, just like Michael used to distract her. I like Cory even more. He's easy to be with and just seems to fit right into our life. It's weird, like Jani and I are both falling in love, but in different ways. When we get home, Jani's respite is here but she is bored, as usual, and asks me, "What are we going to do now, Mommy?" I'm flat down on my bed. Cory puts his hand up and gestures that I stay there.

"Don't worry, baby. You just sleep." *Now, I'm being called 'baby'.* I laugh myself to sleep. Cory entertains Jani and her respite care worker by using his phone to play songs, just like Michael used to. Unlike Michael, he lets me keep sleeping. And I do...for fourteen hours straight. It's the best sleep I've had in years and I wake up to a dream.

CHAPTER 51

MY CORE PACKAGE ARRIVES!

Our Future

Cory is holding my hand as we enter the courtroom. I don't see Michael anywhere but he said he would take Jani to school. They visited Bodhi last night, giving Cory and me more time alone. For two years, I've been celibate, my wants developing slowly. I can't bring in any just guy I'm attracted to because Jani and Bodhi always come first. And in a way, this is a good thing because if I went too fast, I'd probably be setting myself up for a mistake.

*   *   *

Jani and Michael visited Bodhi last night and reported back that, out of nowhere, he pulled one nurse's hair and bit another one. He's throwing feces everywhere and climbing on everything. They had to restrain him, and then give him a PRN to put him to sleep.

"Daddy left me," she says sadly, "but now I have Cory!" She hand-claps.

*   *   *

"I don't want to leave," Cory snuggles into me. It's all so natural. Our bodies fit together like they were made for each other. And for the first time, I don't feel like the mother of a teenage son. I feel like a woman with a man who's really into me. He returns to Seattle November 8th because Bodhi's coming home and I want everything to be exactly the same as when he left.

Every day when I wake up, I feel more of my old self returning. The adrenalin rush I've been on since I first met Michael twenty years ago is waning. I feel like I'm coming off a roller coaster. I'm longing for Cory to come back and he's only been gone for ten days. It's like an eternity.

As promised, on Thursday, November 18th, Cory loads his yellow Penske truck with his belongings and starts driving from Seattle to Los Angeles. He drives seventeen hours straight through to Redding. He sleeps at a rest stop for an hour before driving to Melinda's San Jose home. He takes a shower then heads south, to me.

"Cory! You're back!" He startles me, standing at the bathroom door. I'm fresh out of the shower and jump into his arms. "I missed you!"

"I missed you too, baby." I never liked this infantile term, but right now, in this moment, I feel his love taking me back to a time when I was a baby, soothed in warmth.

*   *   *

Michael is coming to town on the 31st. Bodhi is in the hospital and I'm a mess, but so grateful Cory is here. I didn't realize how alone I've been for so long. All I've heard this past year from Jani is "I want a step-dad."

"I know, but it doesn't work that way."

"Then I'm running away to Ithaca, New York."

"Okay."

Then there's Bodhi. He's so much in need of a father figure. He hangs on Marty, his behaviorist, for guidance. Marty is wonderful. He really provides the type of man I want Bodhi to become. But he will leave soon too, just like all the rest. As much as they *feel* like family, this is still their job and they inevitably move on. All Bodhi has experienced throughout his life is father-figures being there, then leaving him. Worst of all, of course, was when his actual dad left. Cory, or any other man who is a potential partner in my life, will be signing up for not just me, but the Schofield 3.

*   *   *

I update my status on Facebook. It's official. "Cory and I are dating." People are warning me to take it slow. Admittedly, this seems to have literally happened overnight. They don't have to worry because slow is the only way I operate. "I'm definitely taking it SLOW," I reply to all the messages coming in. Meanwhile, Cory's on his computer catching up with the latest news on the Seattle Seahawks.

"Okay, I'm done," I say, closing up my computer as Friday hops onto my bed. Not only do I have two special needs children to take care of but we also have Friday. He doesn't ask for much but he definitely needs to be taken out. Thank God our new apartment complex has a huge dog park in the backyard. I sigh, knowing I've got to get up again, but then I look over at Cory. "Can you take Friday out for me?"

"Sure," he says. Then he does it. It's like he wants to help me.

"Thank you," I say, appreciatively, because I am. The way he does things without any hassle or anger makes me feel like I can just breathe. "Is it alright if I go to sleep now?"

"Ok, sweet dreams because if you let me, I'll talk to you all night."

*   *   *

Later that night, since Bodhi is still at UCLA, I let Cory sleep in Bodhi's bed. It's weird because I've never done this before. Jani's gone to bed and I've already gotten used to staying up a little later than usual while we talk about everything. I feel so much better going to sleep tonight. I'm surprised when I wake up at 4:15 am. I'm sweaty in my nightgown. Usually, I sleep naked, but because of the situation, I don't and I'm sweating. So, I just take it off, forgetting that Cory, not Bodhi, is in the bed beside me.

Then, I start to feel uncomfortable with the situation so I put my nightgown back on again. *Ugh. This is so annoying.* I look over at Cory. He seems to be a little restless in bed. He's clearly not entirely asleep, so I turn to him. "I'm hot. You don't mind if I take this off, do you?"

He shrugs. "No."

"I mean, you can take your clothes off too...if you want." *Did I just say that?*

"Oh, I've been waiting for you to say that." And that's all it takes? I haven't had this for so long. I'm melting inside at his sweetness. "Do you want to be my girlfriend?"

"Yes," I say, without hesitation.

A wide smile spreads across his face. "I want to shout it out to the world that we're dating."

"We can't." I sit up, logic setting back in. "I told everyone I was going to take this slow."

*   *   *

The three of us visit Bodhi at UCLA. Cory doesn't look out of place. He's just a man standing next to Jani and me. But for whatever reason, Bodhi laser-focuses in on him. "Who are you?"

"This is Cory," I tell him simply. Then Jani gives him the Kit Kat bar we promised the day before.

*   *   *

Michael arrives on Halloween night. He knocks on the door, even though it is already open. Melinda always did say he should do this as a sign of respect for my new home. When I open it, he's a bit taken off-guard seeing Cory relaxing on my bed, even though I'd already told him we officially started dating. "This is Cory." I gesture over to him.

"Hey, nice to meet you," Michael shakes his hand, and then matter-of-factly informs me that he wants Jani to spend two nights in the motel with him and they'll go trick-or-treating together.

"Okay." I shrug, a little shaky because Jani's never done this before, but my little Medieval Princess, this year, is fully capable of making her own decisions. I guess he wants to use this to his advantage in front of the judge since this is what fathers without full custody usually do during visitation.

"That's fine. Just make sure that Annette and Alysha know because they'll have to come for her showers."

"Okay." Perhaps he expected more of a reaction from me. It's weird because, if not for Cory, this would have been my first night completely alone in my own apartment. But I have had a lot of unexpected firsts lately.

"Remember, Jani. If you want to come back just call me."

"I know," she says, then leads Michael out the door.

"If I don't see you again…it was nice meeting you."

"You will," Cory says, making me feel even more wanted.

*   *   *

Michael takes Jani out for Halloween night and they go trick-or-treating while Cory and I watch *Ted 2* in complete quiet. No kids to interrupt! It's fun. And it's different. His attention is on me, not anywhere else. It isn't what I've grown used to over the past two decades and I definitely like it.

Visiting Bodhi in the hospital so he has his Minion costume for trick-or-treating around the hospital brings me back to when Jani was there, handing out her "imaginary" rats for candy. She'd wanted to be a "poodle skirt." When we'd gone to visit, her golden locks of hair were wild, black lipstick sliding across her lips and up her cheek, much like the "grown-up" Bette Davis character from *Baby Jane*. I had cried inside, thinking I'd never get my daughter back.

These are the memories I hold onto now, for Bodhi's sake. I know he will get better. Jani did with the right medication, and so will he.

*   *   *

Next, we have Thanksgiving together. We're a new family that came together through God, who used Melinda as our own personal angel. I call Melinda, thanking her for everything she's done for me. Cory has already proposed. Melinda helped find the perfect ring, and it is. How she knew what I would like is beyond me.

"Oh, and remember when Michael told you that 'whales mate for life'? Ask Cory about that."

So, I turn to Cory. "So, whales don't mate for life?"

"No, there aren't many of them so they'll mate with whomever. Penguins mate for life."

When I look back, I'm still sad that our marriage ended but I'm actually happy he has Mia. Without her, he might not still be alive at all and that would be worse for all of us. I don't know why it ended up happening this way, but I guess Michael was always unhappy in our marriage. All I know is that I would rather have him alive than dead and that we were happy together for a long time.

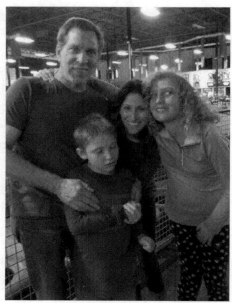

Cory attends a Jani Foundation event with Bodhi, Susan, and Jani.

Too sappy. Whatever it is he has or is, a part of me will always love him. You can't just erase twenty years of life together. There's too much history and there is good inside of that history. But, as with history, life moves on. It's ever-changing, growing in different directions we're not meant to foresee. I don't know what the future holds, but I believe in God and I believe that this is all happening for a reason I cannot comprehend at this moment.

Epilogue

It is Sunday, March 26th, and Michael is visiting the kids, taking them to a birthday party for one of the boys in Bodhi's class. We just got a call from Jessica, a psychologist who saw my latest postings of Bodhi. After 24hospitalizations at UCLA, I am still begging for a Clozaril trial. Jessica offered to reach out to psychiatrists who could help. I'm praying for a psychiatrist to meet with our family and possibly take that next step for Bodhi, and I'm waiting for a call back.

Jani is doing well. Every night, I work to help her catch up on reading and math so she can go into mainstream classes this August. It will be her sophomore year in high school. She is still determined to become a veterinarian and I am determined to give her every opportunity to make this happen.

As for Cory and I, we are a perfect fit. Both Jani and Bodhi have bonded to him. We even set a wedding date for this summer so my father can walk me down the aisle. At 81, he was just diagnosed with Alzheimer's, but not just Alzheimer's. He has Lewy body dementia, which includes symptoms of visual hallucinations, typically of people, children, and animals. Genetics are truly at play here.

The problem our society still faces is the access to medications and their affordability. The mental health system needs to be treated as the serious condition it is. This requires political action for change. We, as the parents of mentally ill/autistic children who will become parents of mentally ill/autistic adults need to receive the appropriate and speedy care NOW! So, this is not the end of my story... it's just the beginning.

This is not the end of my story... it's just the beginning.

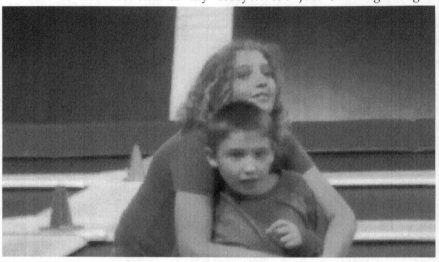

Jani and Bodhi at their favorite trampoline space in April 2017.

PICTURES

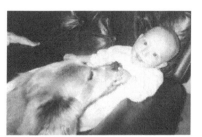

Jani and Honey at our Burbank area apartment.

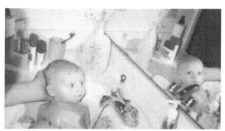

Jani's eyes always told her story.

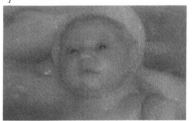

Bodhi's eyes tell his story.

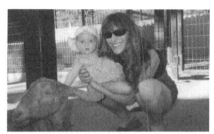

Jani and Susan at the LA Zoo.

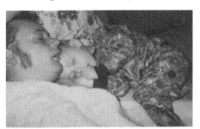

Michael and Bodhi.

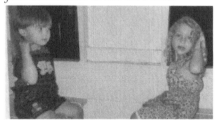

Brandon and Jani at Travel Town.

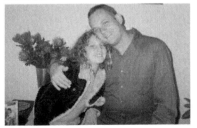

Michael and Jani.

ABOUT THE AUTHOR

Susan Schofield reported news and traffic for local radio and television stations in southern California. She has a BA in Speech Communication from Cal State Long Beach. When her daughter January (Jani) was diagnosed with child-onset schizophrenia at six, she became a full-time caregiver for Jani and two-year-old, Bodhi, diagnosed with autism and intermittent explosive disorder.

Currently, Susan is a mental health care advocate and co-founder of the Jani Foundation, hosting "socialization over isolation" events for special needs kids in the Santa Clarita Valley. Susan has been seen with her family on Oprah, OWN, and TLC. She is now a Producer of Discovery Life's latest documentary on her family "Born Schizophrenic: Big Changes."

You can connect with Susan through:

Email – SusanDSchofield@gmail.com

Facebook – facebook.com/bornschizophrenicbook/

Twitter – @bipolarnation

Because Amazon reviews really do matter, especially for indie authors, please take a few minutes and post a review on Amazon.com. If you notice any errors or omissions, or you see a way to improve this book, please send an email so she can address it. Thanks!

Other Books

By Michael Schofield
Contributions From Susan Schofield

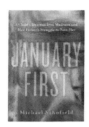

A *New York Times* bestseller, *January First* captures Michael and his family's remarkable story about mental illness. In the beginning, readers see Jani's incredible brilliance followed by early warning signs that something is not right, Michael's attempts to rationalize what's happening, and his descent alongside his daughter into the abyss of schizophrenia. This battle included countless medications and hospitalizations, allegations of abuse, despair that almost broke their family, and, finally, victories against the illness and a new faith that they can create a life for Jani.

Born Schizophrenic is a semi-sequel to *January First*. While it continues their story up through early 2017, it also covers the earlier years, but from Susan Schofield's perspective.

By Liza Long (Foreword)

Liza Long is the mother of a child with bipolar disorder. When she heard about the Newtown shooting, her first thought was, "What if my son does that someday?" Her emotional response to the tragedy, published as "I Am Adam Lanza's Mother," went viral, receiving 1.2 million Facebook likes, nearly 17,000 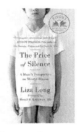 tweets, and 30,000 emails. In *The Price of Silence*, she takes a devastating look at how we address mental illness, especially in children, who are funneled through a system of education, mental health care, and juvenile detention that leads far too often to prison.

By Liz Long (Editor)

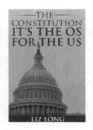

The Constitution: It's the OS for the US explains the US Constitution in terms modern Americans can understand: computer terms, not legal ones. (An OS is a computer Operating System, like iOS for Apple devices.) For example, the President is like Power-Point: not a lot of power per se, but a lot of power to persuade and indirectly cause people to do things.

OMG! Not the Zombies! Book 1 is a zombie series for those who like a good zompoc story but not gory descriptions of what happens. This is a full-on zompoc series about what happens when a group of teens brings home an ax with the zombie virus on its edge, but it tries to keep a sense of humor even as the undead take over the elementary school playground.

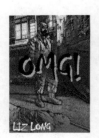

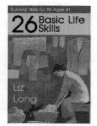

Survival Skills for All Ages #1: Basic Life Skills teaches basic skills other books assume you know including following a recipe, dressing for the weather, food safety, cleaning, basic first aid, and simple sewing. From situational awareness and trusting your instincts to preserving food and safe knife use, the skills this book covers are useful in real life *and* emergencies.

Made in the USA
San Bernardino, CA
12 July 2018